"*Sandplay Wisdom* is a gift to sandplay therapists and Jungian analysts, as well as to all of us who care about psyche and life. Sandplay needs wisdom, so as for our daily life. This book embodies the nature of the Kalffian-Jungian sandplay method: the way of life."

– **Heyong Shen, City University of Macau; President,
Chinese Society of Analytical Psychology**

"*Sandplay Wisdom* represents an extraordinary legacy of two leading sandplay therapists based on four decades of personal clinical experience. It contains a wealth of theoretical considerations incorporating Jungian psychology, attachment theory, and neuroscience, among others, touching on how this therapy works, how it came into existence, evolved and in particular how it can be used to benefit both children and adults in distress, including those who suffer from trauma. A variety of case studies illustrate the theory and bring it alive. The book will not only be a fundamental companion for students and practitioners of sandplay but reaches out to anyone who wants to understand more deeply the self-healing potential inherent in an approach which integrates body, mind and relationship."

– **Martin Kalff, PhD; sandplay therapist, ISST**

"*Sandplay Wisdom* documents four decades of collaboration between Friedman and Rogers Mitchell, pioneers in sandplay therapy. This volume encompasses the foundations of sandplay, how it heals, ego development, childhood issues of loss and trauma, working with adults, transference and countertransference; it is rich with case examples. This book is a rich resource of their creative and original work which has influenced sandplay therapists over the years and will continue to have a significant impact for the future of sandplay therapy."

– **Audrey Punnett, PhD, RPT-S, CST-T/ISST; Jungian analyst;
Vice President of the Americas, International Association of
Sandplay Therapy; past President, Sandplay Therapists of America**

"With great admiration and respect, I enthusiastically recommend Harriet and Rie's new book. This book covers important aspects of sandplay therapy, and, most impressively, many sandplay cases are given to illustrate the main points. This is a valuable book for professionals who teach sandplay and for those who are interested in advancing themselves in sandplay work."

– **Grace Hong, PsyD, LP, ISST-TM**

Sandplay Wisdom

Sandplay Wisdom provides key concepts for understanding and using sandplay therapy effectively, distilling insight from more than four decades of experience. Rie Rogers Mitchell and Harriet S. Friedman provide both core principles and hard-won practical tips to deepen understanding of sandplay therapy for both experienced and novice practitioners.

The principles presented provide key insight into many important therapeutic dimensions, including childhood trauma, archetypal life stages, age and gender issues, transference and countertransference, as well as sandplay with both adults and children. The book is illustrated with case material and images from real sessions throughout and provides invaluable guidance on working with clients in a vast range of contexts.

This important book will be essential reading for all sandplay therapists in practice and in training. It will also be of great interest to practitioners, academics and scholars of play and arts therapies.

Rie Rogers Mitchell, PhD, ABPP, is Professor Emeritus in educational psychology and counseling at California State University, Northridge. She studied with Dora Kalff, the founder of sandplay, and has served as president of the International Society of Sandplay Therapy and president of Sandplay Therapists of America. She received the 2015 Kalff-Bradway Award for recognition in Sandplay Therapy.

Harriet S. Friedman, MA, LMFT, is a Jungian analyst and certified sandplay therapist practicing in Los Angeles, California. Inspired by studying with Dora Kalff, Harriet became a founding member of Sandplay Therapists of America. She is a member of the International Society of Sandplay Therapy, and received the 2016 Kalff-Bradway Award for recognition in Sandplay Therapy.

Sandplay Wisdom

Understanding Sandplay Therapy

Rie Rogers Mitchell and Harriet S. Friedman

Routledge
Taylor & Francis Group

LONDON AND NEW YORK

First published 2021
by Routledge
2 Park Square, Milton Park, Abingdon, Oxon OX14 4RN

and by Routledge
52 Vanderbilt Avenue, New York, NY 10017

Routledge is an imprint of the Taylor & Francis Group, an informa business

© 2021 Rie Rogers Mitchell and Harriet S. Friedman

The right of Rie Rogers Mitchell and Harriet S. Friedman to be identified as authors of this work has been asserted by them in accordance with sections 77 and 78 of the Copyright, Designs and Patents Act 1988.

All rights reserved. No part of this book may be reprinted or reproduced or utilised in any form or by any electronic, mechanical, or other means, now known or hereafter invented, including photocopying and recording, or in any information storage or retrieval system, without permission in writing from the publishers.

Trademark notice: Product or corporate names may be trademarks or registered trademarks, and are used only for identification and explanation without intent to infringe.

British Library Cataloguing-in-Publication Data
A catalogue record for this book is available from the British Library

Library of Congress Cataloging-in-Publication Data
A catalog record has been requested for this book

ISBN: 978-0-367-62627-3 (hbk)
ISBN: 978-0-367-62628-0 (pbk)
ISBN: 978-1-003-11000-2 (ebk)

Typeset in Times New Roman
by Deanta Global Publishing Services, Chennai, India

Contents

Acknowledgments

Our professional and personal partnership over the past 40 years has been a rich and rewarding experience. We were pleased that Susannah Frearson at Routledge appreciated the importance of publishing this culmination of our work together. We are indebted to her for recognizing the potential for this book and supporting our endeavor. We are grateful for Sushmitha Ramesh and others at Routledge who worked on the book.

Deep appreciation is warranted for the dedicated efforts on so many levels by Gita Morena, PhD, CST-T, and Rex Mitchell, PhD. Without their steadfast and wise participation in this book, it would not have been born. We are grateful beyond measure for their assistance throughout the process.

We are also grateful for the community that has supported us over the years and has welcomed our thinking and innovation in the field. In particular, we want to acknowledge Sally Suggat, Jill Kaplan, Marion Anderson, Judy Zappacosta, Betty Jackson, Janet Tatum, Audrey Punnet, and Joyce Cunningham for their continued enthusiasm, partnership, and engagement.

Harriet extends her special thanks to the Los Angeles Sandplay Group, including Gloria Avrech, Janet Blaser, Joan Concannon, Antionette Eimers, Susan Frankel, Lori Tyler, Gail Gerbie, Adele Lutrell, Debbie Mego, Barbara Moreno, Nancy Paul, Shawnee Smith, and Marci Loftin.

Rie sends her special thank you to her many clients who informed and inspired this book.

Both of our families have been our true cheerleaders over the entire arc of our work together. We are thankful for the support of our husbands, children, and grandchildren.

And to all the Sandplay Therapists and fellow travelers to whom we have presented all over the world.

Preface

For four decades we both have been studying, teaching, writing together, and presenting our work with sandplay therapy to clinicians and students around the world. Widespread interest in this work moved us to publish two previous books, *Sandplay: Past, Present, and Future* (1994) and *Supervision of Sandplay Therapy* (2008), several chapters in other books, and many articles in *The Journal of Sandplay Therapy*. The mystery and energy of sandplay has enriched our lives far beyond anything we could have imagined. It appears that sandplay has also captivated the imagination of many clinicians throughout the world. To our surprise we have been asked to teach in many countries, including Australia, Brazil, Bulgaria, Canada, China, Germany, Holland, Hong Kong, Israel, Italy, Japan, Korea, Macau, Poland, South Africa, Spain, Switzerland, Taiwan, and Uruguay, as well as many parts of the US.

During these experiences across many languages and cultures, we have been impressed with the shared common core of understanding and experiences with sandplay. It is one of the few therapeutic techniques in which language is unnecessary for understanding the expressions of the psyche. The nonverbal, symbolic nature of sandplay provides a vehicle for the unconscious to let itself be seen and known. Within this complex world, sandplay offers a unique opportunity to view universal, archetypal patterns, as well as to observe the unfolding development of the individual psyche. It has become a cross-cultural method that is increasingly practiced worldwide.

Sandplay has helped each of us to be able to work with a deeper and fuller understanding of the psyche, allowing us to connect with both the conscious and the unconscious aspects of what is going on in the psyche. Using nonverbal sandplay together with verbal therapy has opened us to a whole new level of understanding of the psyche that can image intense and sometimes long-forgotten emotional affects within individuals. We have come to see how different parts of individuals are revealed, including those not evoked by verbal methods alone.

We have learned that sandplay deepens and accelerates the therapeutic endeavor. As the mind and body interact in the sand, the imagination is stimulated and creativity is evoked. While this process is occurring, verbal complexes, dreams, personality, and life problems are thrust into consciousness. We have observed that sandplay encourages the individual to work with this creative technique, which enables healing.

And now, after so many years, we have even more respect for the silent essence that is established between ourselves and the sand players. This relationship sustains the work through challenging times. As C.G. Jung states, "The inner voice is the voice of a fuller life, of a wider, more comprehensive consciousness" (2014, p.184).

In this book, our desire is to share with you the highlights of what we think are the most valuable insights to help your study and experience of sandplay therapy. This book is a culmination of our passionate interest and work with sandplay, what we have learned to focus on in our years of working with this technique, and the many transformations that have occurred for our clients – as well as for ourselves. Working together for these many years on this material, the energy between the two of us has grown and also inspired us to share the insights we have gained. We have written this book with our deep appreciation for the many people who have used, written about, and added to our knowledge about this extraordinary technique. We hope this book will deepen and enrich you on your sandplay journey.

Reference

1. Jung, C.G. (2014). *The development of personality*. Routledge. (previously published in 1954 as *Collected Works of C.G. Jung*, Vol. 17, Princeton University Press)

Chapter 1

What is sandplay?

Sandplay was developed by Dora Kalff, a Swiss Jungian-oriented therapist, in the 1950s. Sandplay is a powerful nonverbal and symbolic form of therapy that gives both child and adult clients the opportunity to portray, rather than verbalize, feelings, experiences, and internal states often inaccessible and/or difficult to express in words. Sandplay therapy facilitates the psyche's natural capacity for healing and can be used in conjunction with traditional verbal therapy.

A basic premise of sandplay therapy is that the psyche possesses a natural tendency to heal itself, given the proper conditions. Similar to how our physical wounds heal under beneficial conditions, the psyche also has an instinctual wisdom that emerges when left free to operate naturally in a protected environment.

The aim of sandplay therapy is to activate healing energies at the deepest level of the psyche by using miniatures and a sand tray to reflect the client's inner world. By this activity, and through the experience of free and creative play, unconscious processes are made visible in a three-dimensional form, much like a dream experience.

Thus, sandplay provides a vehicle for the unconscious to let itself be seen and known. Through the process of playfully creating sand trays, individuals often retrieve lost memories, work through trauma, discover unrealized aspects of the personality, and integrate parts of their personality – thus leading to a sense of greater balance, wholeness, and an enriched, more satisfying life. The nonverbal, symbolic nature of sandplay makes use of the natural language of the unconscious and provides a needed balance for today's extraverted, technological, and outer-focused everyday world. Sandplay promotes a more natural, balanced, and integrated way of life.

The sandplay method is deceptively simple. The therapist creates a free and protected environment in which the client can relax and let his or her internal state be accessed and expressed. Using sand, water, and miniature objects within a shallow box (28 ½" × 19 ½" × 3"), which is painted blue on the bottom and sides, the client creates a three-dimensional picture (i.e., a concrete manifestation) of his or her inner imaginal world.

Some children, mostly those eight years old or younger, create dynamic pictures that are constantly in movement until coming to rest when the child moves on to something else in the therapy room. Older children and adults often comment about their scene. However, interpretations and discussions about the trays by the therapist are not initiated until after a series of trays has been created over time (This is called a *sandplay process*). It is important that the sandplay process remains at a nonverbal, instinctive level, rather than a cognitive, intellectual place, so that the unconscious can continue to be accessed without client concern about what the therapist has said or might say about the sand picture. In this way, sandplay helps honor and illuminate the client's internal symbolic world and provides a place for its expression within a safe container, i.e., the tray filled with sand.

Upon completion of a sandplay picture during a therapy session, the client may make comments about the scene, which are usually recorded by the therapist.

After the client leaves a sandplay session, the therapist photographs the scene. This picture is then stored with the client's other sandplay photos, awaiting completion of the sandplay process. Finally, after the sandplay process is complete, the client and therapist may view the photographs and reflect on and decipher the content of the trays and the process itself. Providing such a window into the unconscious deepens understanding of the individual psyche and provides a framework for future verbal therapy.

Five important characteristics define the Kalffian-Jungian sandplay method:

1. The therapist must provide a *free and protected space* for the client to be able to create a picture in the sand tray, with no interpretation of the tray and not much verbal interaction as it is being made. It is the therapist's nonverbal acceptance of the images used in the tray that is essential. This period of relative quiet helps both the client and therapist stay attuned to what is being created in the sand and concentrate on what images emerge in the tray

2. A sandplay process consists of the trays that the client creates over time. Usually the tray-making process leads toward natural development or a sense of unification

3. Delayed interpretation: In the sandplay work, therapists try to follow the client's natural way of being, rather than leading the experience. During the tray-making process, there is relatively little verbal exchange between the client and therapist. Of course, if a client asks where a particular miniature is located, the therapist responds, but the therapist does not make comments or ask questions during the process. This quiet space helps the client and the therapist stay attuned to what is being created in the sand and does not interfere with the client's feelings or images that are being created in the tray. The miniatures on the shelves are the symbols that speak the language of the unconscious and provide indications of the client's inner drama. Later, after the entire sandplay process comes to a natural conclusion, the therapist and client may agree to view and discuss the trays. This is often a powerful event; the verbal and nonverbal join together

4. After a scene has been created in the sand tray, it is not taken apart in the presence of the client. The scene is a statement of the client's psyche. Taking the scene apart in the presence of the client is disrespectful and could be a damaging experience. Normally, a picture of the scene is taken after the client leaves the therapeutic session; the scene is then dismantled

5. Sandplay is part of a larger therapeutic experience that may include other therapeutic methods, for example, ongoing verbal therapy about concrete life events, unconscious material such as dreams and fantasies, and verbal interpretations by the therapist. Only one part of what is going on in therapy is the creation of the sand pictures; that part, the nonverbal, is a deliberate regression into the symbolic level of the psyche

The most important aspect of using sandplay effectively is the preparation and personal development of the individual therapist. Becoming an effective sandplay therapist is an engaging and interactive process that requires developing the ability to receive, facilitate, and understand the profound experiences and imagery that this medium can evoke. Comprehensive clinical training, involvement in one's own personal therapy, and experience as a practicing therapist are all important. It is recommended that therapists interested in sandplay training read about and take courses in sandplay, Jungian theory, and symbolism, and complete their own sandplay process in order to enhance understanding of the therapeutic process. Further, a sandplay consultation group experience can be very helpful.

In 1982, Dora Kalff officially founded the International Society of Sandplay Therapy (ISST). Since that early period, sandplay has spread worldwide with official national associations in China, England, France, Germany, Italy, Japan, Switzerland, and the United States. In order to be a Certified Sandplay Therapist (CST), candidates must successfully complete a series of educational requirements, write papers, involve themselves in their own personal sandplay process, and participate in group and individual supervision. To become a Certified Sandplay Therapist-Teacher (CST-T), and thus be certified to teach and supervise others, additional requirements must be met, including co-teaching with a certified teacher and presenting cases before an evaluative audience.

In addition to Kalff's *sandplay* approach, the term *sand tray* is also used to refer to the use of miniatures in a shallow box filled with sand. However, s*and tray* is a generic term that is used more broadly to include such applications as: (a) using sand trays for research or as an assessment instrument, (b) using trays with more than one individual (e.g., families, couples, and groups), (c) situations where a therapist is not present, or (d) when the therapist is an active participant in a directive or interactive capacity.

Because sandplay is one of the few therapeutic techniques in which language skills are not necessary for understanding the expressions of the psyche, it has truly become a cross-cultural method that is now practiced therapeutically worldwide. Within this ever-shrinking world, sandplay offers a unique opportunity to view universal, archetypal patterns, as well as to observe the unfolding development of the individual psyche.

Suggested reading

Kalff, D. (1980). *Sandplay: A psychotherapeutic approach to the psyche*. Temenos Press.
Mitchell, R.R., & Friedman, H.S. (1994). *Sandplay: Past, present and future*. Routledge.
Weinrib, E.L. (1983). *Images of the self: The sandplay therapy process*. Temenos Press.

Chapter 2

How does sandplay heal?

A basic premise of sandplay therapy is that the psyche possesses a natural tendency to heal itself, given the proper conditions. Similar to how physical wounds heal under certain conditions, the psyche also has an instinctual wisdom if left free to operate naturally in a safe and protected environment.

According to Jungian theory, the Self is located in the unconscious – the place of wisdom – and is the central ordering principle of the entire personality. The ego is located in the conscious part of the psyche, which is the center of consciousness, but less than the whole personality.

The connection between the Self and the ego is an important concept in Jungian psychology – for when the Self and ego are in relationship (i.e., in communication), then the individual is living closest to his or her own actualized state and thus feels more balanced and alive. Sandplay can be an effective means of evoking and nurturing the vital bridge between the Self and ego. Why is that?

The unconscious uses symbols as its language. It is a shared human experience of having one's unconscious expressing itself symbolically through dreams, art, play therapy, and other imaginative activities. In essence, the unconscious talks in symbols.

In sandplay, the sand provides a stage where symbolic objects can be placed. The tray itself provides a *temenos* (the Greek word for "container") for the safe containment of these energies. Thus, sandplay provides a safe space for the unconscious Self to be seen and known by the conscious ego (through the use of symbolic miniatures). Said in another way, sandplay acts as a conduit or bridge that facilitates communication between the Self (in the unconscious) and the conscious ego.

How does this happen in sandplay? What is it about the sandplay experience that facilitates communication and enhances healing? Let us consider the sandplay process and how each part of that process works together to provide healing or transformation. All of the parts are important, but what is even more important is that these parts work together to form a gestalt in which the whole is greater than the sum of the parts. That whole leads to communication and ultimately to healing.

The following attributes of sandplay are important in facilitating and enhancing healing:

1. **Turning the focus inward**: Putting one's hands in the sand, shifting and moving it around, is a kinesthetic experience that moves the focus away from the outer world – the conscious mind – and inward to the body, and ultimately to one's internal realm. In everyday life, we usually do not focus on our internal world. Having an experience with our body helps us move inside ourselves. So, the client should first touch and feel the sand before selecting objects to be placed in the sand

2. **Activating healing energies**: As the individual scans the collection of miniatures, some items seem to be invested with a magnetic draw. The client's attention is pulled to them, and they are chosen because of the unconscious symbolic meaning that is projected onto these objects. Once this internal energy field has been established (between the client's psyche and the symbolic miniatures), activating the healing aspects of the unconscious becomes possible

3. **Giving expression to the unconscious**: The sandplay materials (i.e., the sand, miniatures, and sand tray) offer an opportunity for unconscious psychic components – previously held in check, now striving to break through – to be unconsciously and symbolically revealed and expressed in the sand scenes. This process is similar to recording dreams: the unconscious is activated in sleep, expressed through symbols, and then written in a dream journal

4. **Creative stimulation**: In participating in this expressive process, the client has the opportunity to sense the stirring and emergence of his/her own creative healing powers and become aware of something bigger and more inspiring than him/herself. The experience of creating a sand picture is occasionally accompanied by an extraordinary numinous moment, similar to having a profound insight or deep spiritual awakening. Such a moment happens when the Self is touched. This special moment is often chronicled in the sand picture itself

5. **Presence of the other**: The unconscious moves freely to deeper levels as the sandplay experience unfolds in the presence of another, the therapist, who mirrors and accepts, without judgment or analysis, what the psyche has presented. The therapist creates the free and protected space while acting as a witness of the process. Having a witness results in a bigger impact than just creating trays by oneself – another dimension is activated

6. **Integrative viewing**: The viewing of the sandplay creation in the presence of the therapist, promotes increased consciousness and integration of unconscious material by bringing it into tangible three-dimensional form. Interpretation is unnecessary and hinders the unfolding process.

   These above six attributes are critical. A seventh step adds to the experience, particularly with adults, but is not essential with children

7. **Review and reflection**: Some time after the completion of a series of trays, healing is enhanced through having the client and therapist reflect on the sandplay process and analyze the trays together. Moving understanding closer to conscious awareness continues the vital link between the Self and the ego

Case of Brett

This case illustrates many of these attributes. Brett, a seven-year-old boy, suffered from early separation caused by the divorce of his parents. He was one of many children who are caught in the changing family systems of today's society, like so many children seen in therapy.

Brett's mother and father were divorced when he was 18 months old. Their relationship had been difficult during the marriage and continued to be difficult after the marriage broke up. Brett divided his time between their two homes. Both of the parents were remarried. Brett had not received enough emotional support early in life to make sense of the many disruptions in his world, especially the rage of his parents, which went on around him before and after the divorce. His parents were too immature, themselves, and too taken over by their own primitive anger to think about their young son and give him the support and understanding he needed. From early on, Brett felt overwhelmed and confused about what was going on around him. Therefore, part of Brett's personality remained in a state of confusion, panic, and despair.

As a small boy, his connection with his mother lacked closeness. She was working, and Brett had been left for long periods of time with a variety of caretakers. Even when he and his mother were together, it seemed to him that she was unable to provide much emotional structure or containment to protect him from the chaos that surrounded him.

The parents had decided on a joint custody arrangement. Both parents said that Brett seemed to have adjusted well to that arrangement. Every weekend he made the switch from one household to the other. He was an ordinary student at school and got along well with his sister, who was two years older. However, after one year of moving from one house to another every week there were signs that Brett was struggling with this arrangement.

In school, Brett's teacher had noticed his attention had begun to diminish. Also, the Sunday evening switch from one parent's house to the other was now accompanied by more clinging and crying, following which he would quickly withdraw to his room – especially when his parents would lapse into fights around him. The parents had a long history of loud screaming arguments that frightened Brett.

The idea of bringing Brett for treatment first came up when he began having trouble falling asleep and would cry out for more comfort. His pattern was to return to sleep, only to awaken several more times, asking for more and more soothing. This behavior so worried his mother that she contacted a therapist. She was concerned about suggesting treatment for Brett to his father. His father was against any kind of psychological intervention. He believed that Brett should just "toughen up" and that his mother should set firmer limits and stop comforting him at bedtime.

So, the subject of therapy for Brett was dropped, but his disturbing behavior continued, particularly when he was at his mother's house. It wasn't until his father and new family had endured many sleepless nights with Brett that Dad finally agreed to treatment. However, Dad made it clear that Brett's treatment was going to be according to his rules and on his terms: (a) the therapy was to be limited to nine months – no longer; (b) Dad was to interview and have final approval of any therapist; (c) the therapist was not to have any "secret contact" with his ex-wife; he was fearful that the therapist might be in collusion with her and that he would become the scapegoat.

The therapy then began. Brett participated mainly in traditional, play therapy treatment. He also created eight sandplay scenes during his nine months in therapy. Either Brett or the therapist would suggest doing a tray. These eight sand scenes illustrate a meaningful healing progression.

His sandplay trays are not very different from most boys of his age. However, in the child-like naturalness of his sand scenes, it is possible to feel the powerful energy of his psyche that moved him toward wholeness. Watching this case unfold demonstrates that the healing experience for Brett comes directly from relating to his fantasy play in the sand.

It is the play and the interchange between internal fantasy images and concrete use of images in the sand that activate the internal healing energies that reside within. Sandplay gave him the opportunity to express his feelings and fantasy. This experience offered the opportunity for him to visibly express formerly repressed feelings and to make them available to be seen, freeing up energies that can be used constructively.

Figure 2.1 (Tray 1)

Brett made this first sandplay during his second session. I see it as Brett's way of communicating his state of inner disorganization and chaos. Often an initial tray depicts the outer reality of a situation and to me this tray depicted both Brett's inner and outer realities.

At this point, Brett was in a very alienated state. He was flooded with primitive material, as represented by the fighting dinosaurs and scattered marbles. The discord between the animals mirrors the discord at the core of his being. The vicious fighting that had surrounded him as he grew up is depicted in the tray. He so often felt at the mercy of these angry affects that could, and did, overwhelm him. He was unable to speak of these powerful emotions, yet he needed to have them seen by me. His ego was clearly overwhelmed.

This tray was created with a lot of activity on Brett's part – lots of moving objects around. His later trays are more like pictures, but this particular one is a dynamic tray – typical of many trays done by children under eight years of age. Children under that age are more likely to use toys actively, moving them in the tray (sometimes quite dramatically), often speaking or making noises for the miniatures. This tray was created in that way.

In his play therapy sessions, Brett was very active and distractible, jumping from activity to activity. I felt his anxiety in the sessions, which he was acting out through this hyperactive behavior. Some of these early sessions were particularly exhausting – not easy to get through.

Note that this first tray has no internal boundaries; the contents spill out all over, much like our time together in play therapy. I wondered what I was observing during the sand play sessions. Was he a child with ADD? Was I watching his acute anxiety? Was this state an agitated depression? Based upon this tray, I concluded that his behavior was communicating anxiety. Even though there are no internal boundaries, the contents contain intense focus, intense detail, and cohesion that might not occur with an ADD child. The fighting between his parents continued to be a dominant force in his life. As a result, he always seemed to be struggling to contain an ongoing chronic anxiety. He simply could not relax.

Even though there are three sets of dinosaurs that continue to fight, there are now two dinosaurs differentiated from the others, alone and not fighting. When Brett finished this tray

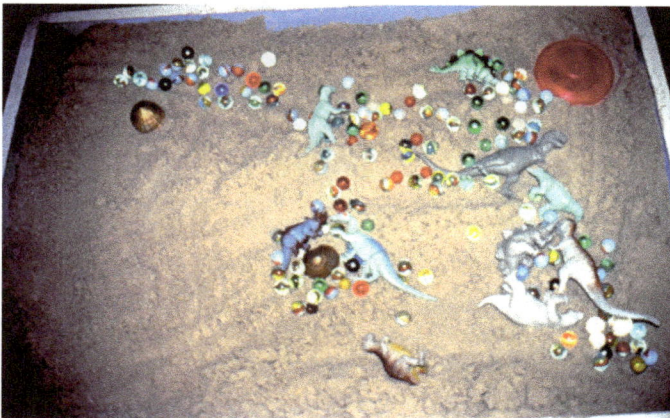

Figure 2.1 Tray 1

he said, "These dinosaurs just don't know how to stop trying to kill each other; they need my help." Then he took the watering can and doused two of them slowly and carefully with water. It was as though he was beginning to experience himself not just as a passive onlooker but also as someone with some power to cool things off.

I was pleased to see the few golden shells that he used. Gold represents a highly prized substance, also a superior quality, and it is associated with the sun as well as the earth. I saw the circular quality of the small red disc in the upper right corner as an indication of wholeness and energy within him. Perhaps he was trying to bring about a centering and a safe place from the considerable anger and chaos that surrounded him. I saw both the golden shells and the red disc as positive and progressive indicators in this mainly destructive, chaotic tray. I wondered if and how these two symbols might manifest in future trays. I hoped that the healing energies in this tray would be supported in therapy, so that they could guide him in coping with his destructive family situation. These symbols of wholeness in this early tray encouraged me, even as the considerable chaos gave me pause.

Figure 2.2 (Tray 2)

I was pleased to see Brett make more space in the tray. His beginning ability to move the sand indicated his readiness to use inner resources. I knew that in moving the sand in the tray, Brett was also attempting to enlarge or restructure his inner world, a task that would be crucial for him in coming to terms with his life situation. Dr. Ruth Bowyer's research found moving the sand to be an indication of a child's ability to utilize their inner resources in a creative way. She also suggests this is an indication of above-average intelligence (Mitchell & Friedman, 1994, p.67).

He was beginning to use vegetation. I was happy to see some new growth here. The inclusion of plant life is related to an inner sense of potential for psychological growth, in contrast to the starkness of sand trays that connote feelings of lifelessness. Brett's own potential for growth was now becoming visible.

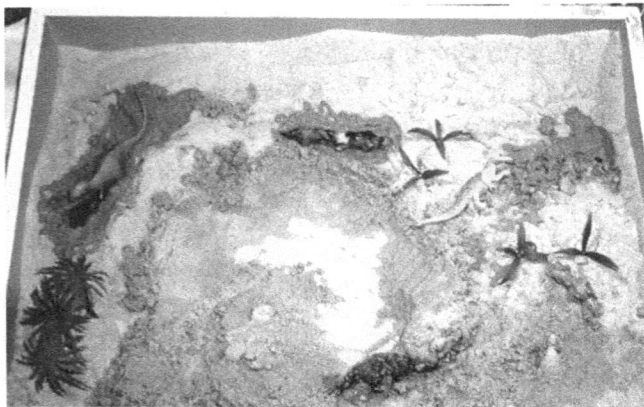

Figure 2.2 Tray 2

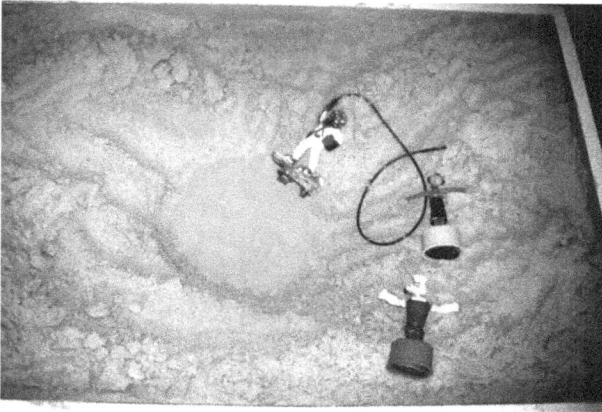

Figure 2.3 Tray 3

Figure 2.3 (Tray 3)

In this tray Brett took a lot of time to smooth the sand and make a large clearing, so the blue bottom of the tray could show through. It was as though he was now able, at long last, to make more space for himself in his world. Of course, that had been a major problem for him; his parents' fighting had taken over. Brett couldn't find enough space of his own while growing up. However, here he is able to finally begin the necessary separation from his parents. He uses a deep-sea diver, perhaps a figure that depicts himself diving into the depths, and leaves behind Popeye and Olive Oil, who may be representing his Mom and Dad.

Figures 2.4, 2.5 and 2.6 (Tray 4)

This tray reminded me of one of those transition trays, where there are pieces of the old situation but also pieces emerging of a new organization that is coming together. There are several new pieces here, but they are not all connected or even standing up yet. Generally, when I see prone figures in a tray, they alert me to a particularly deep level of wounding that has been experienced and express how very difficult it is to find a solid, grounded position from which to stand up and meet the situation. This sand picture conveyed the devastation that Brett had endured. The roads don't go anywhere and neither does the tunnel. Even the devil is prone.

However, on the right side something very important was beginning to happen. Brett put together three pieces of a mountain/bridge and connected them to each other (**Figures 2.5 and 2.6**). I saw his ability to choose these separate parts of the mountain and then put them together with the bridge as an important metaphor for the internal construction making place in his own center.

The bridge was to become a very important symbol for Brett – a symbol of reconciliation and the ability to relate, contact, and communicate with others while also keeping his separateness. For him, having the ability to bridge helped him make the ongoing transition between the families bearable. After he made this tray, I never heard complaints from the parents that he was upset when he left to go to his father's house or returned to his mother's.

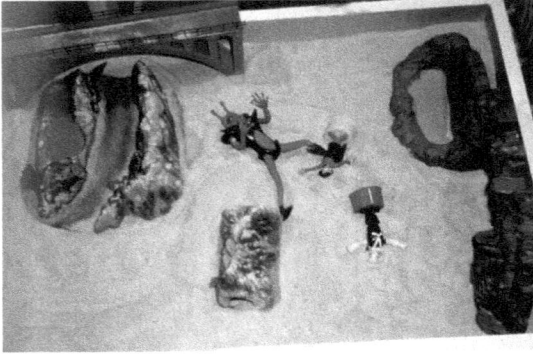

Figure 2.4 Tray 4

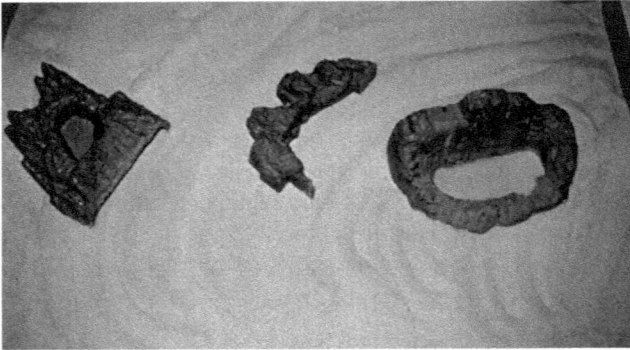

Figure 2.5 Tray 4 detail

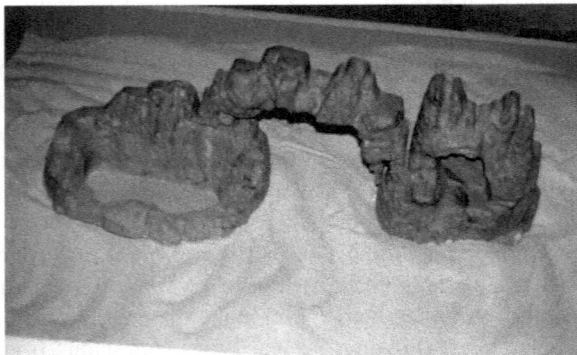

Figure 2.6 Tray 4 detail

By this time in the treatment, after about four months, Brett was sleeping much better. According to his teacher at school, he was starting to come alive socially and, much to everyone's surprise, was taking a new interest in books and has become an avid reader.

Figure 2.7 (Tray 5)

Again, Brett made space in the tray for himself. He used the figure Pluto the dog to depict himself, even while the fighting continues. He chose to put Popeye and Olive Oil on top of a castle, separated in space but together in the same house. Perhaps the castle is the beginning of a container for the parents. This is common with children doing sandplay: the repeated use of the same figure or figures in a series of trays. Pluto (representing Brett) stands separate on the mountain/bridge, which Brett once again put together in the tray. Notice now he has a more objective and separate view, as he looks over the entire situation by himself. It was striking that this separation and coming together was possible; even as the dinosaurs continue to fight, the new growth and his separateness continues.

In school, Brett's teacher had reported to the parents that he was now the best reader in the class. Brett was very proud of himself, as were both his parents.

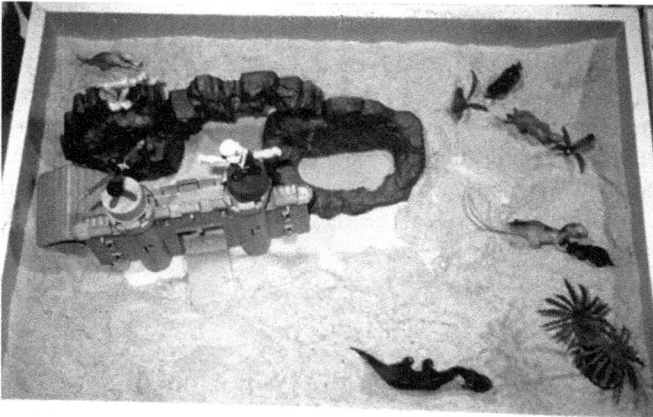

Figure 2.7 Tray 5

Figure 2.8 (Tray 6)

Here Pluto (Brett) continues to stand separate from Popeye and Olive Oil. While the fighting does continue, it was lessened in this tray. Now Pluto looks toward the oasis, no longer turned toward Popeye and Olive Oil. Although nothing in Brett's outer reality had changed, his behavior appeared more settled and independent. Water continued to be a strong theme for Brett; this time, perhaps it was a symbol of an internal life-giving and nourishing source.

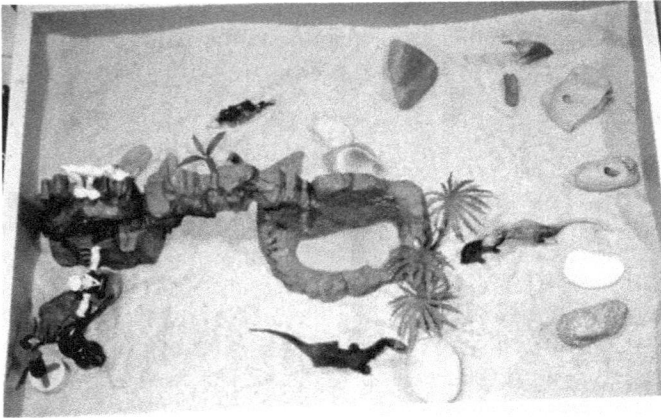

Figure 2.8 Tray 6

Figure 2.9 (Tray 7)

Brett had one more month of therapy left. He had been working hard each week to put together a rocket ship model. It took a lot of patience, plus careful reading and following of instructions for him to complete it. We were both very proud of this accomplishment and he had been looking forward to using it. He told me many imaginative scenarios of how the rocket ship might be used when he had finished it; one of them was to use it in a sandplay.

Here, the mountain/bridge structure continued to be used, and the new rocket ship he had proudly made was present. I was both pleased and surprised to see the reuniting of the family in the center. The outer situation had not changed, but here in the depiction of his internal state, a profound resolution had occurred.

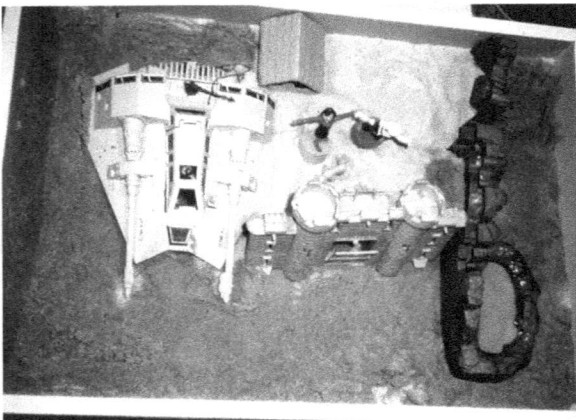

Figure 2.9 Tray 7

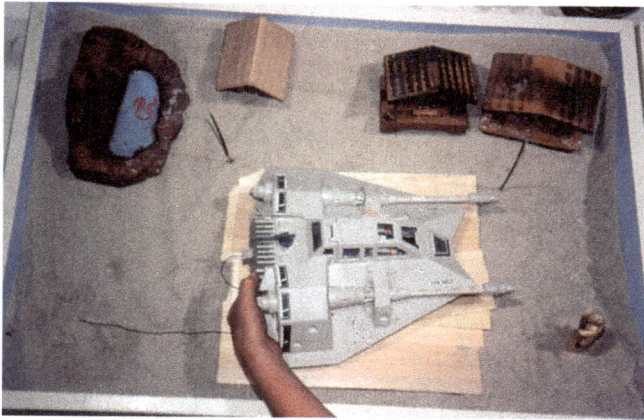

Figure 2.10 Tray 8

When Brett finished putting the pieces in the tray, he took a long time watering down the outside edge as though to calm it all down. Perhaps it was to christen and launch his new self into the world. A new, single house has emerged, perhaps finally a place for him to experience himself outside of the conflicted environment. Also, now holding hands, Popeye and Olive Oil have become the agreeable internal parental images he had never experienced in his outer life. There was great intensity in creating this tray.

Figure 2.10 (Tray 8)

This final tray was created in Brett's last session. It was now the end of the nine months that his father had given us to work together. Brett and I were both very aware that this would be our final meeting. It felt to me as though this sandplay was created in almost a sacred atmosphere.

Before Brett began to create this tray, he asked me to put two pieces of incense in the tray and light them for him. He began by putting in the three houses. I wondered if now there was a separate space for mother, father, and himself. He used the pool section from the mountain he had used so many times and carefully filled it halfway with water. Inside the pool he placed a small orange snake. (The snake is a symbol of transformation; snakes shed their skin with regularity). I believe Brett had gone through a transformational experience himself.

He asked me to get some of the wood he had seen piled outside my office to use as a platform from which he could launch his rocket ship. His psyche was preparing him for a new separation, not only from me, but also from his warring parents. After I gave him the wood, he put the ship on the launching pad and said he wanted me to take a picture as he was about to lift the ship off and that I wouldn't have the whole story right if I didn't have his hand in the picture. Brett said "this *Star Wars* figure is going to climb on board to keep him company so he wouldn't be alone." I saw that his growth had provided just what he needed – Yoda, a wise, archetypal companion.

Brett had moved from a state of isolation, fear, and confusion to one of confidence, clarity, and strength – he was now ready to take off. This young boy, like many children who do sandplay, was able to find his way to his internal home once he was free to play imaginatively and be himself. He was able to move from a state of alienation to an internal feeling of his own wholeness.

This series of sand trays shows a profound reorganization of Brett's psyche. In his outer world his parents' difficult relationship continued unchanged. However, the development of Brett's inner security created a foundation for his emerging and separate selfhood to take hold. It was a pleasure and moving experience to have been able to follow and accompany him on his particular journey.

Reference

Mitchell, R.R., & Friedman, H.S. (1994). *Sandplay: Past, present and future*. Routledge.

Chapter 3

Archetypal life stages

This chapter analyzes sandplay scenes created by three adult females, each of whom was in the midst of a biological life transition: (a) before menstruation begins, (b) the coming of the blood, and finally (c) the ending of menstruation. These three different stages often serve as "building blocks," defining change and/or possible transformation and initiation to another level of physical and psychological consciousness.

Recognizing that these are universal themes often allows women to move through these life-changing processes feeling connected to the feminine mysteries. These transition times are larger than merely personal events; they are also archetypal events, and it helps to understand that these events are far beyond our own control. This gives us comfort and support as we are thrown out of our ordinary lives and into the larger and more chaotic times of transition, reminding us that we are only a small link in the great chain of life.

The particular images of these three women's experiences are similar to those that have been manifested since the beginning of time. There are traces of similar healing images in shamanism, as well as in all indigenous cultures. Thus, sandplay stimulates the imagination to create personal images in a way that connects each of us to the larger archetypal world. That is exactly what all three of these women were able to do.

Jung (1971, p.66) writes about how the imagination works, "It functions like a lamp and not a mirror." Therefore, instead of the mind being passive when images emerge, there must be active participation on the part of the individual in this image-making experience.

In today's culture, initiatory rites are almost non-existent and life transitions, such as beginning womanhood (e.g., menstruation), are often not acknowledged in a positive way. This makes these and other life transitions more difficult to accept and experience.

Eric Neumann (1973, p.186) described it this way, "In modern man [where] collective rites no longer exist ... psychic disorders are frequent ... not only in childhood, in puberty, in marriage and mid-life ... and in the hour of death. All these stages in life were formerly numinous points at which the collective intervened with its rites; today, these are often times of psychic illness and anxiety for an individual, whose awareness does not suffice to enable him to live his life".

Indigenous cultures seem better able to celebrate life's transitions than our own culture. Their rites usually include one or more older individuals, who had been through the experience themselves and can offer empathic guidance and support through this time of change, guarding the person against dangers, such as depression, confusion, and overwhelming feelings.

In the following three cases, sandplay, within the therapeutic relationship, activated the instinctual wisdom of the psyche and provided the space necessary for initiatory life experience. For each of these three women something from a deep archetypal source knew that a meaningful rite must be performed to acknowledge the passage from one life stage to another.

Case 1: Jasmine's initiation process

Jasmine's mother brought her for therapy because she and her husband were concerned about Jasmine's withdrawal, anxiety, and possible depression. The case of this ten-year-old client illustrates transition into adolescence.

Her mother described Jasmine as a sweet, bright, creative, and complicated child, who has a low frustration tolerance and either gives up or cries when frustrated, yet she does very well in school.

Jasmine's relationship with her father was one of distance. Her father was a busy, powerful, and publicly acclaimed man, who was often away from home. He was also a warm and captivating individual, but he was just not available to Jasmine. She wished that she could spend more time with him. His passion was swimming, and Jasmine enjoyed that with him.

According to her mother, Jasmine denies that she worries and is protective of her mother. However, just as therapy began, Jasmine had a dream about a hunting shark. In the dream, Jasmine jumped into the water to tell her mother that the shark was coming, even though her mother was not in the water.

Over a period of 10 months of weekly therapy sessions, Jasmine created 26 sandplay pictures, 15 of which are included in this chapter (they are numbered as Trays 1–15 for convenience).

Figures 3.1 and 3.2 (Tray 1, two views)

This tray contains an amber rock, turtle, bone with arms and legs (rectangular figure), totem pole (reflects family history among the native tribes in western Canada and Alaska), two Kachinas (Hopi deities), ants, and three snakes.

In this first sandplay, Jasmine holds the sun (solar energy) over her tray. It seems that her new energies (as represented by the baby) need to be sheltered within the protection of the tepee from the assault of the sun in order to grow and develop in a healthy manner. I felt this was an unconscious message to me that I needed to move carefully (dimly). Two Indian

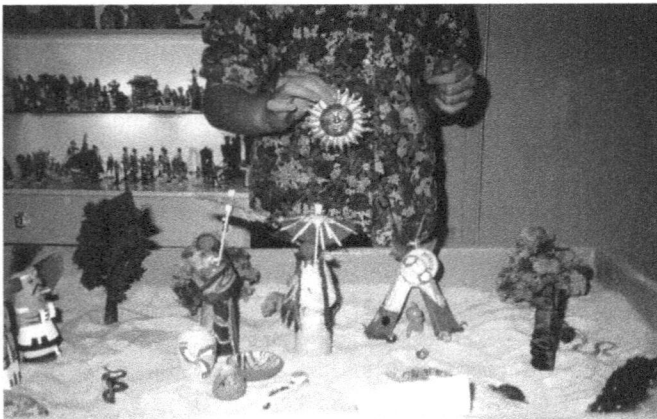

Figure 3.1 Jasmine's Tray 1

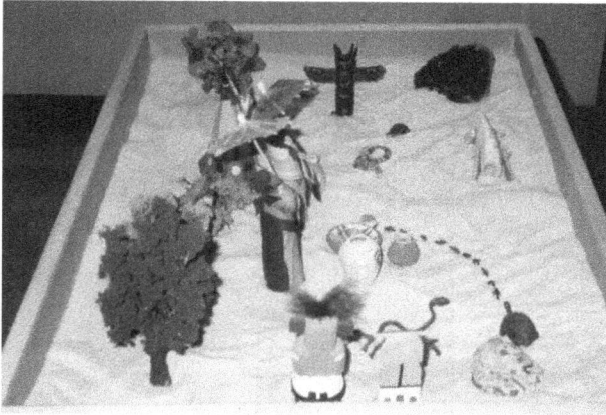

Figure 3.2 Jasmine's Tray 1, different view

women (a mother and daughter) are standing close together, holding umbrellas to protect themselves from the sun's heat. At their feet are vessels for holding food and water; however, these are empty. She initially placed food in the vessels and then removed the food, suggesting to me the possibility that she may be unready, as yet, to begin the journey, particularly with the sun shining so brightly.

In viewing the tray from the side, the close proximity of two Indian women is apparent, which supports observations made by Jasmine's mother. Her mother was worried because Jasmine seems too attached to her. She said, for example, that Jasmine often intuits and then expresses her (the mother's) feelings and ideas instead those of her own. Her mother also felt uncomfortable because Jasmine never expresses any anger toward her. Instead, Jasmine tries to protect her and appears to feel responsible for her mother's feelings.

In this tray, it seems that Jasmine's energies have been activated; the totem poles and Kachinas are thought to evoke ancient ancestral energies. The trees suggest a potential for growth and development. The snakes indicate activation at a primordial level in her psyche and, according to Kay Bradway (1980), snakes can be a bridge to the beyond.

This is a girl who needs to start living her own life and begin preparation for her later initiatory experience. She feels she needs to take care of her mother, which prevents her own individual development and forward movement. At the same time, she idealizes her father, but he is unavailable to help. She needs to move into her own mode of being and to cut the psychic umbilical cord.

Figure 3.3 (Tray 2)

One month later, in her second sand tray, Jasmine created a sacred atmosphere. The feminine Buddha takes center stage, suggesting that the feminine has been activated. According to Jasmine, this Buddha is in a Japanese museum and is guarding the treasure: the egg, candelabra, and crown. I thought to myself at that time, "these three elements are necessary for Jasmine's growth."

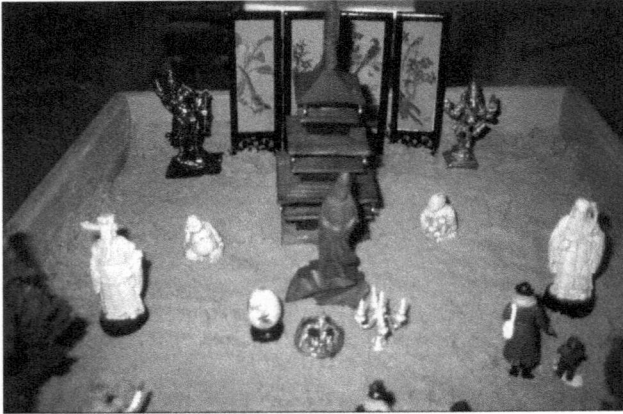

Figure 3.3 Jasmine's Tray 2

Like the baby sheltered within the tepee in her first tray, Jasmine's egg needs shelter and protection in order to grow. Certainly, the human egg needs the sanctuary and darkness of the womb to develop. With care and protection, the egg signals the possibility of birth with a new point of view.

The crown in the tray may herald Jasmine's ability to rise above her present situation. The crown is often a symbol of spiritual evolution; i.e., victory of a higher principle over the base principle of the instincts. C.G. Jung (1967a, p.190) considered the crown to be a par excellence symbol, for it suggests the possibility of reaching the highest goal in evolution – spiritual evolution. Jung said, "Those who have conquered (themselves) win the crown of eternal life." A candelabra symbolizes spiritual light, understanding, and salvation. When I observed these three symbols being placed in front of the protecting feminine goddess, I knew that Jasmine had the potential to move forward onto her own individual path.

Figure 3.4 (Tray 3)

In her third tray, two weeks later, Jasmine created an age-appropriate scene where she surveyed the landscape of her own childhood, in contrast to the adult rendition in the previous tray. She placed herself on a bridge, objectively overlooking the area. I saw here evidence of the development of a more reflective or objective view or, in other words, an observing ego.

Jasmine was a high achieving, adult-like child. Her mother described her as an "old soul." Seldom had Jasmine let herself be a child, freely playing and enjoying a park, such as the one she created in the sand tray. However, her park is not entirely carefree; a threat is evident in the background, symbolized by the masculine cannons. A fence is placed between the park and the outer world. Is this fence for secrecy, privacy, protection, or something else?

After the emergence of the feminine goddess in the previous tray, there was now more room for her to examine herself with more objectivity. However, room for movement (where the bicycles are moving) remains limited. Yet a snake from the first tray and flowering trees from the second tray hint at the possibility of transformation and new developments.

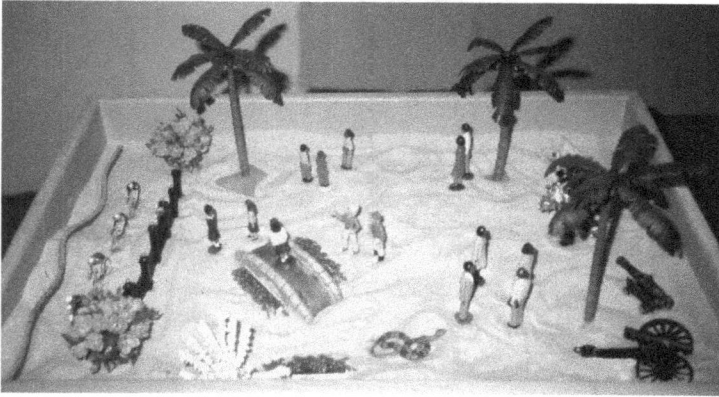

Figure 3.4 Jasmine's Tray 3

Figures 3.5 and 3.6 (Tray 4)

In conjunction with the previous tray, Jasmine's fourth tray created two weeks later is an excellent demonstration of the developmental process with its movement back and forward. After exploring her more child-like world in the last tray, Jasmine's psyche now moves in a more expansive direction. Here the crown appears again, placed on the ground, seemingly waiting for the feminine to claim it.

According to Jasmine, the crown is part of a procession. The king, princess, and queen are walking toward the crown and the prince consort. Now, perhaps, there is more room for movement. Jasmine states that the queen needs many guards (lining the path). She shows me where "the normal people are standing (behind the fence) and watching." It appears that her psyche is heralding the possibility of her newly developing feminine uniting with the masculine on an equal basis – not as afraid or sheltered from the masculine. The golden coach is ready and waiting.

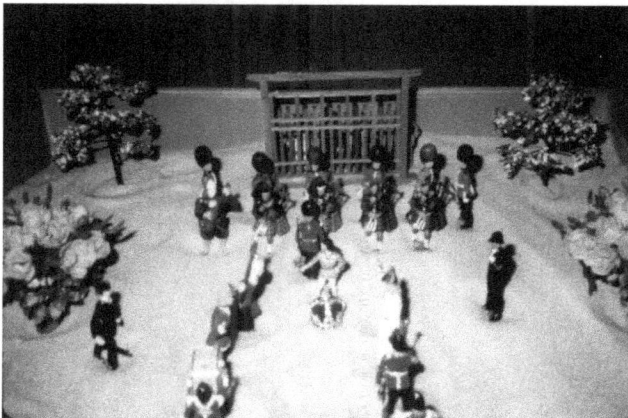

Figure 3.5 Jasmine's Tray 4

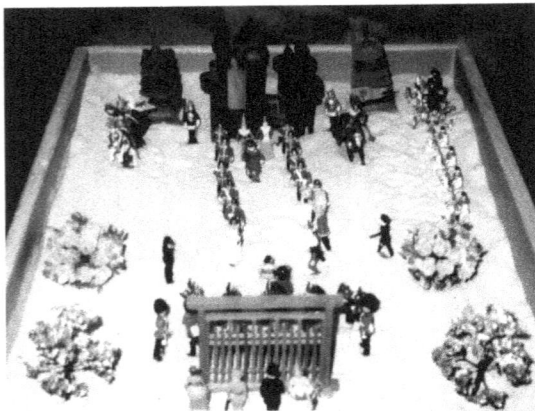

Figure 3.6 Jasmine's Tray 4

Figure 3.7 (Tray 5)

Two weeks later, Jasmine creates a tray she names "Boston 1774: the Boston Tea Party." In getting ready to create the scene, she changes her standing position so that we are face to face. She wants me to view the whole tray as she makes it, so I can witness her act of emancipation. It is quite an achievement for this heretofore, obedient girl to show anger or aggression in her tray. However, in the form of rebellious Americans throwing tea into the harbor, she is communicating her own rebellion. She needs an older woman observer (the therapist), to witness her natural adolescent rebellion.

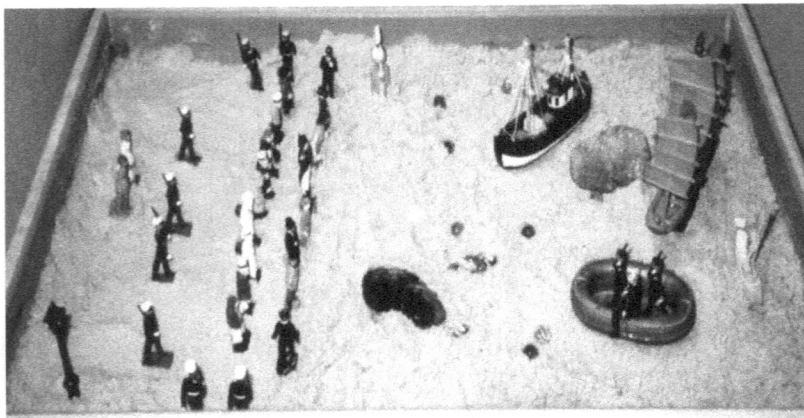

Figure 3.7 Jasmine's Tray 5

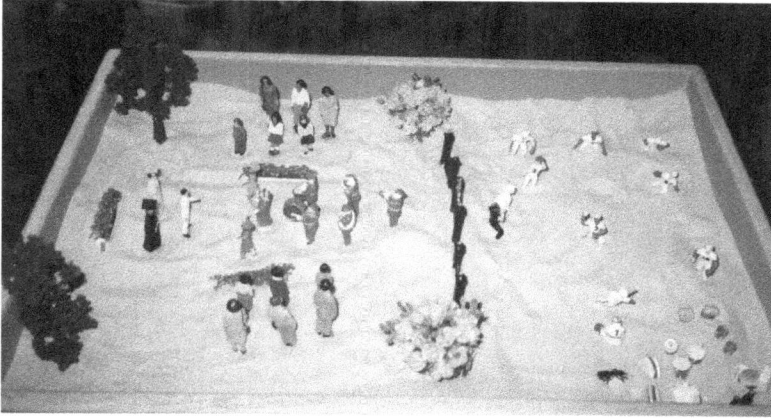

Figure 3.8 Jasmine's Tray 6

Figure 3.8 (Tray 6)

After showing her age-appropriate rebellion in the previous tray, on the same day she makes room for even more age-appropriate play (baseball) and for nutrition from age-appropriate food: hamburgers, fries, and sodas. On the other side of the tray, she portrays a graduation ceremony, suggesting readiness to move into the next phase of her new development.

Figure 3.9 (Tray 7)

Now, two weeks later, there is even more room for an expansive experience in what Jasmine calls "The Wax Museum for Children." Here, people are looking at child-like figures with an

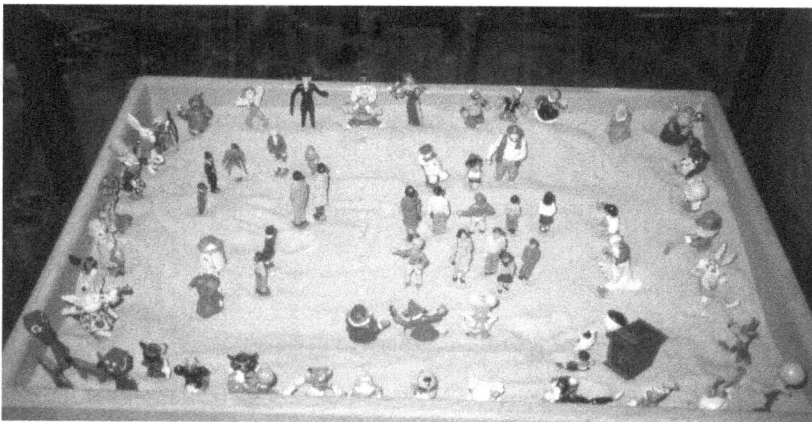

Figure 3.9 Jasmine's Tray 7

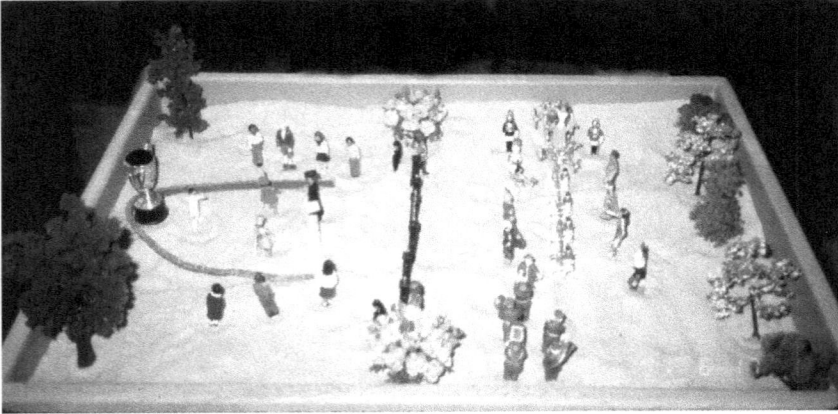

Figure 3.10 Jasmine's Tray 8

objective ego. I thought to myself, "Oh, it is as if Jasmine is looking back with an objective stance at the childhood she has now left behind but preserved in a museum."

Figure 3.10 (Tray 8)

In this tray, created three weeks later, the feminine becomes a central figure again. This time the figure is an even more evolved feminine, a queen rather than a princess, and appears in a form closer to her own identity (rather than an Asian goddess form). Jasmine says that this is the Queen of England coming to California with her carriage and private guards. I thought, "Something new is arriving and announcing itself." On the left side of the tray is a golden trophy with a girl in white standing in front. Jasmine told me that she was going to be in a spelling bee in a few days and hoped to win (She didn't win, but still did very well).

Figure 3.11 (Tray 9)

One month after the arrival of the queen in the previous tray, a celebration takes place in a sacred and separate place. In this tray, a new element is introduced – fire – denoting that a new level has been reached. I could feel Jasmine's excitement as she lit the red candles. The guards are present again, protecting her sacred place and secret egg, as she calls it. The egg is in the center of the tray, between the girl in pink and the golden Buddha. I wondered to myself if the secret egg and red candles herald her future menstruation and increased maturity.

Figure 3.12 (Tray 10)

Three months later, a celebration is held again. The egg has matured and babies are born. She places additional babies in the surrounding tents, suggesting more potential is yet to emerge. The snake energy follows and helps her. Two women from her first tray appear again, but now

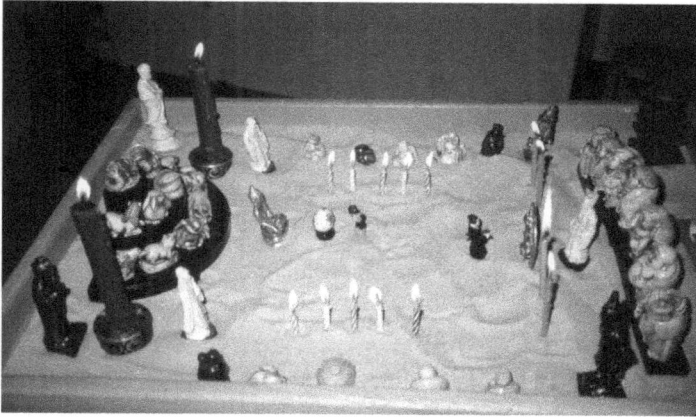

Figure 3.11 Jasmine's Tray 9

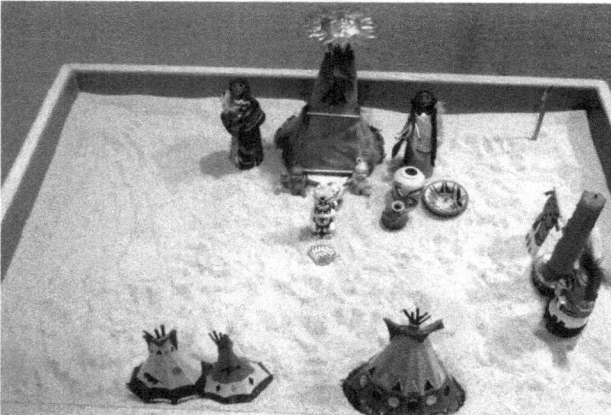

Figure 3.12 Jasmine's Tray 10

they are more separated. This time the open containers hold something she calls "Previous." The Kachinas are prominent, along with a red candle. She then asks me to take a picture.

Figure 3.13 (Tray 11)

This tray, created on the same day as Tray 10, retains the major miniatures in their same places. However, Jasmine moves the sun from the top of the largest teepee to the ground. Then she positions two babies in front of the tepees, adds several small miniatures, including gold ones, and places 28 round blue gems throughout the tray.

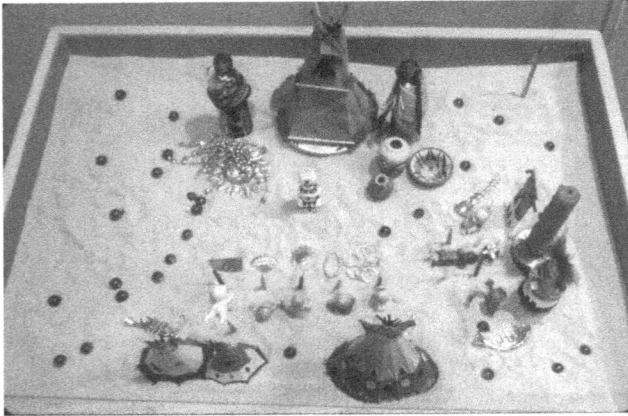

Figure 3.13 Jasmine's Tray 11

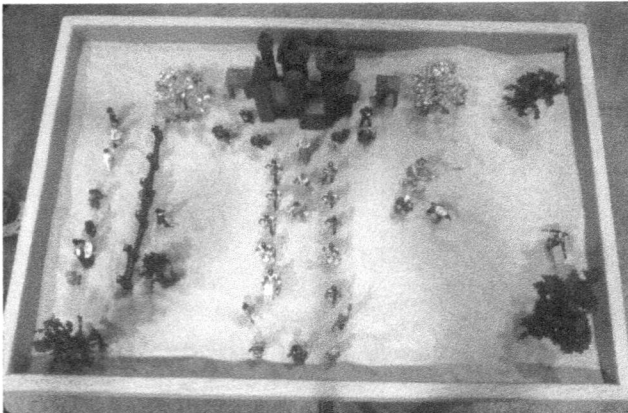

Figure 3.14 Jasmine's Tray 12

Figure 3.14 (Tray 12)

The king and queen, arriving from the castle, are walking between two rows of soldiers. On the left side of the tray, people are watching from behind a fence.

Figure 3.15 (Tray 13)

On the same day as Tray 12, Jasmine created this tray while standing at the shorter side of the sand tray. This is a very symmetrical picture. Much green vegetation is spaced throughout the tray, suggesting even more growth. A fenced area in the top quarter of the tray contains two beds and objects of value and is framed with flowering bushes. She places a clay vessel near the left front. Several animals, plus a peacock, are arranged evenly around the tray. Then,

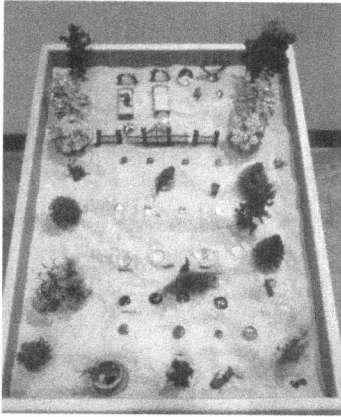

Figure 3.15 Jasmine's Tray 13

she creates five horizontal rows, each with four evenly placed round gems: red, blue, clear, smaller clear, and green rows from front to rear.

Figure 3.16 (Tray 14)

Around the top, right, and bottom sides of the tray, Jasmine places many miniatures. These include three tepees, two oriental paper umbrellas, several figures, a clay pot, a flat basket with gold rings lying on top, and much green vegetation. On the left side of the tray is a figure in a yellow canoe, moving directly toward the top of the tray, with sand contoured to resemble a river. The sand, in the center rectangular space of the tray, is arranged to suggest horizontal movement. Near the right side of the clear space is a female riding a white horse,

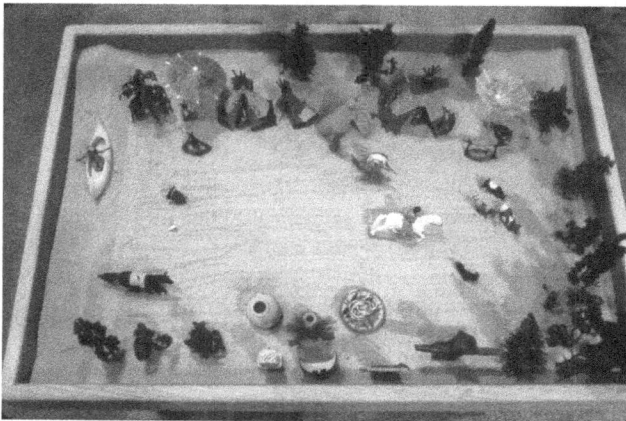

Figure 3.16 Jasmine's Tray 14

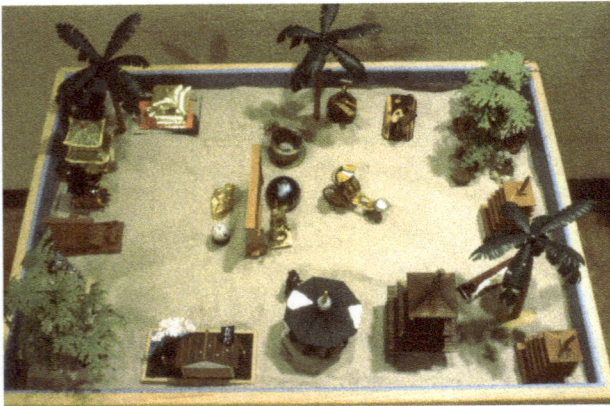

Figure 3.17 Jasmine's Tray 15

moving to the right. Above the horse is a figure dressed in red, pointing a gun at the horse and rider. At the bottom left corner of the clear space is an unridden black horse with a yellow blanket on its back. Also, there are several small animals in the clear space.

Figure 3.17 (Tray 15)

Jasmine's final tray is a beautiful, organized picture. She places green trees near each corner, followed by five pagodas and a well. In the center, two gold objects and two spheres bracket a screen. After she created this scene, she expressed that she felt ready to end therapy.

All of Jasmine's trays were carefully organized, especially her last ones. Jasmine had one more session where we viewed and discussed pictures of her sandplay trays. She told me that she now felt less anxious and freer to be herself in the outside world.

Case 2: The coming of the blood

Fran, who was 16 (nearing 17), had not yet begun to menstruate. Her sandplay experience helped her make the transition from her childhood state into a fuller and more developed sense of womanhood.

Fran's mother had worked with a colleague of mine and was worried about her daughter. Fran was fully developed physically, yet she still wasn't menstruating. The family doctor suggested hormone shots to bring on her period; however, something inside Fran's mother rebelled against this medical approach. Mother's former therapist suggested that perhaps sandplay might reveal some hidden blockage in her daughter's development. Soon after this, Fran's mother called me for an appointment for her daughter.

Fran's parents were divorced, and she was living with her mother, step-father, and older sister. In our work together, we talked quite a bit about her life, sorting out her feelings about her parents' divorce, as well as her school concerns, driving license, and friends – but never about how she felt about not yet menstruating. The deep issues that were expressed in her trays were rarely spoken of directly between us.

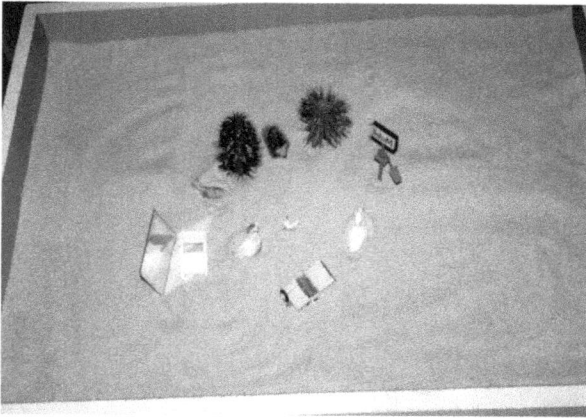

Figure 3.18 Fran's Tray 1

In our work together over nine months, Fran created sandplay pictures periodically but not every week. As she worked in the sand two dimensions were experienced: (a) the conscious, social, and verbal level, and (b) the nonverbal, unconscious aspect. These two levels of communication ran concurrent with each other and were vital and complementary parts of her rite of passage.

Figure 3.18 (Tray 1)

Fran's first sandplay was created during our third therapy session. I was struck by the dry and lifeless feeling of this tray, the lack of connection in her placement of the animals, and the mirroring of what had gone on in her own family. It was so sad to see the empty chair placed next to the mirror. Perhaps this represented her own mother, close but not able to mirror her. All the objects in the tray are close together; however, they are not related to each other and face outward into space. The green flourishing trees felt hopeful, indicating (or suggesting) the possibility of a renewal. The porcupine looks toward the gasoline pump in the center, perhaps, like Fran, looking toward me to help her connect to her own depths for nourishment.

Figure 3.19 (Tray 2)

Some weeks later, Fran created this tray. I thought this sandplay was a portrayal of her present state, with yet deeper feelings now activated. Although there is conflict present in this tray, it felt to me that there was more energy – a relief to me. An internal battle is going on and a military commander is in control of the whole scene. I saw the military trucks and fighting soldiers reflecting the destructive aspect of her life situation.

In the center, a helicopter is trapped in a tree. Her development was stuck, as was the helicopter. Her natural growth, in the form of the tree, was indeed established. Here is the portrayal of her natural feminine growth trapped in a masculine dominated struggle. I wondered to myself how she could get out of this powerful masculine entrapment.

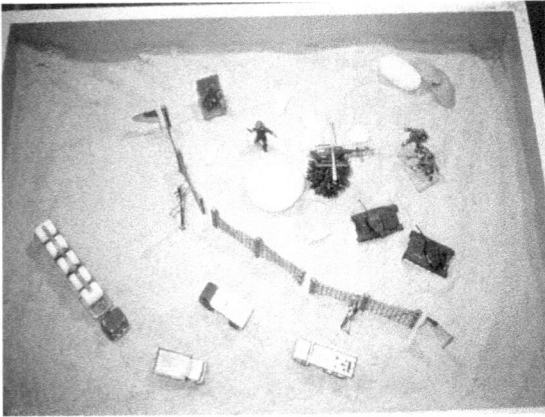

Figure 3.19 Fran's Tray 2

Figure 3.20 (Tray 3)

The three spiders perhaps represent the three females in her family, including herself. The little girl sitting alone at the table is similar to how Fran adapted within the family – staying young and distant and, therefore, out of the family conflict in order to feel safe. All this is happening as the clock is ticking; time is going by. I silently wondered, "Was she going to get it together and perhaps menstruate soon?"

Around this time, Fran was anxious about another rite of passage, one that would move her closer into the adult world – qualifying for a driver's license.

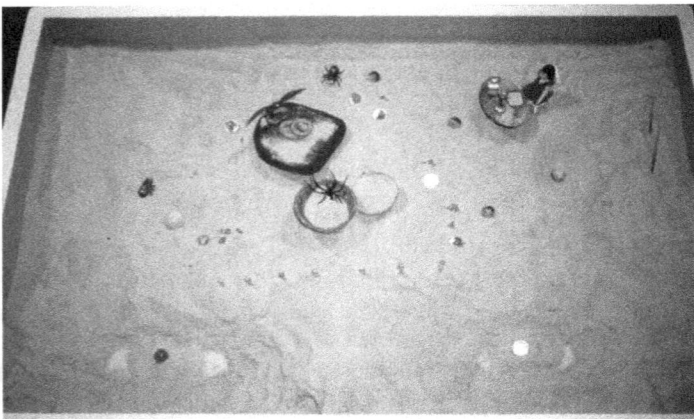

Figure 3.20 Fran's Tray 3

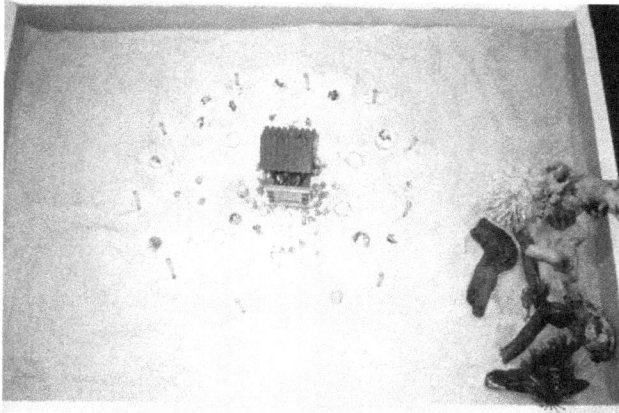

Figure 3.21 Fran's Tray 4

Figure 3.21 (Tray 4)

She said, after she created this tray, "I'm walking out of a dark forest and I'm real surprised to find this well here." In this sandplay, Fran comes upon her own center, symbolized by the well, the deep source within herself. The old, gnarled branches and dying trees indicated to me that Fran was letting go of the innocence of her early childhood state in which she had been living. Hopefully she is now getting ready to move on into the next phase of her development.

One month following this tray, Fran completed her driving lessons and passed her driving exam without difficulty. In the following months, she displayed more energy and self-assurance, as well as being more reflective about her early life and beginning to envision her possible future.

Figure 3.22 (Tray 5)

In a more reflective mood, Fran created this picture in total silence. When she finished she said, "I guess that's her. All alone and leaving now." I realized that she was talking about the imaginary child that she was in the process of leaving.

As time passed, Fran began finding the strength to become more outspoken in her family and thus more involved.

Figure 3.23 (Tray 6)

Fran put an incredible amount of energy into making this sand picture. The mirrors balance the most precious jewels of her feminine self. One mirror is full; the other enables her to reflect back on this powerful experience. The golden shell at the mouth of this vaginal opening represents the deep value to which she now feels connected. The red disc is the ability to menstruate – I hoped. The lighthouse indicates the path she is clearly on. The fences are the old restrictions she has put behind her.

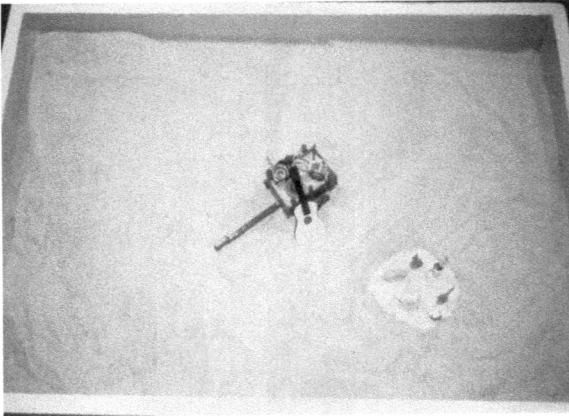

Figure 3.22 Fran's Tray 5

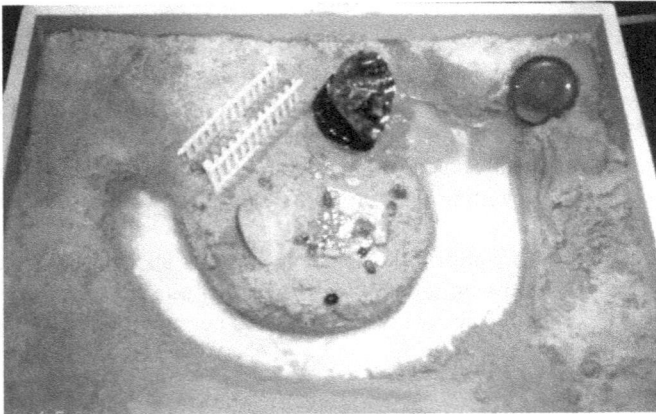

Figure 3.23 Fran's Tray 6

Figure 3.24 (Tray 7)

A month later, Fran silently walked into my office and sat down. She put her head down and didn't speak. Nothing I tried to say seemed to touch or move her. I had never seen her so totally withdrawn and silent. Then she moved slowly into the sandplay room when I asked her if she would like to do a sandplay. I felt concerned about this very dark and solitary place into which she had so suddenly and unexpectedly dropped.

First, she made a clearing in the center of the tray. Into it she slowly dripped red and black candle wax. It was very compelling to watch her do this in total silence. I was sitting on the edge of my seat as she worked. Finally, she looked up at me with her eyes filled with tears that were spilling down over her cheeks. She then announced to me, "I got my period at school today." She then blew out the two candles and ran out of the office without another word.

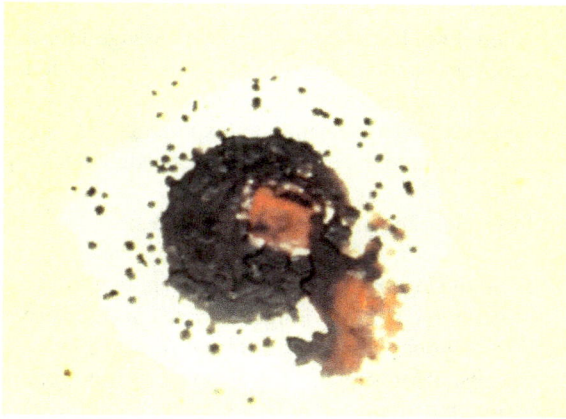

Figure 3.24 Fran's Tray 7

Her tears, her simple words, "I got my period at school today" accompanied by what her hands were able to express in the sand – all came together – from some deep archetypal source within her – she created a much needed, but uniquely her own, initiation rite in the sand. I certainly felt honored and deeply touched to have been able to be a witness to this numinous rite of passage .

Figure 3.25 (Tray 8)

I saw the driftwood, like her old child-like identity, was now discarded. The pelican – the nourishing, self-sacrificing mother watching close by – points to Fran's new connection to the positive aspect of the mother archetype. In her use of the starfish, an animal able to

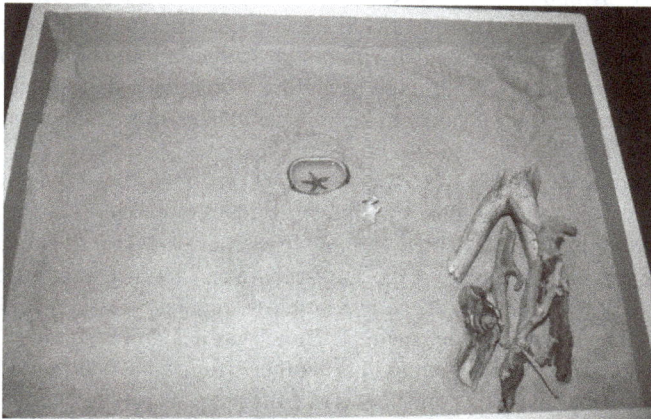

Figure 3.25 Fran's Tray 8

regenerate and grow a new limb when the old one has been injured, confirms to me that Fran has also been able to restore parts of herself.

With this final tray our work terminated. Fran had clearly made the passage into womanhood. I felt it was her new found consciousness and connection to her own self that allowed her the freedom to move away from the extroverted, materialistic lifestyle and now be able to come into her own maturity. I also believe it was the sandplay experience that supported Fran through the rite of passage that brought her into the experience she needed: her very own blood mystery initiation.

Now a quote from Jung (1967b, p.114) about the movement of our lives:

> Our life is like the course of the sun. In the morning it gains … in strength until it reaches … high noon. The … steady forward movement no longer denotes an increase, but a decrease … Thus our task in handling a young person is different from the task of handling an older person … It is a great mistake to suppose the meaning of life is exhausted with the period of youth and expansion; the afternoon of life is just as full of meaning as the morning … its meaning and purpose are different.

A menopausal woman: Ending the flow

From Fran's story, in the morning of her life, to Rachel, a menopausal woman in the afternoon of her life. Sandplay helped Rachel find the unique meaning and purpose of the final stages of the blood mysteries.

Rachel was on a month-long sabbatical from a mid-western state hospital where she had been a nurse for over 20 years. She was in Los Angeles at the Jung Institute when she noticed a brochure describing a workshop I was giving featuring sandplay. She called me for an appointment.

We then began to work several times a week when she was in Los Angeles. Later, over a ten-year period, she made many more trips to Los Angeles to continue our work together, eventually moving to Los Angeles. In our time together, verbal therapy and sandplay went on side by side. Both of these processes worked together to support her journey.

When we first met, Rachel was in her early forties. She came into therapy not because of any disturbing "menopausal" symptoms. She never even mentioned anything about menopausal issues until almost the last part of our work. She came into treatment because she had a feeling of emptiness and that her life seemed without any direction. Rachel had never married. But the most immediate and upsetting issue in her life at that time was a long-term relationship with a married man that didn't appear to be going anywhere more than what was happening at the moment.

When Rachel was 2 years old, her mother, who was a mere 16-year-old, gave Rachel to her own older unmarried sister, some 14 years older, who lived in a town close by.

Rachel's father had left her mother and herself soon after Rachel was born. By the time Rachel was two, her mother was overwhelmed by the conflict between her own needs and her toddler's needs. Over time, Rachel's mother visited less and less frequently, so Rachel lived with her aunt for the next 15 years in a nearby town until she was a senior in high school. At that time she returned to live with her mother and her mother's fourth husband for a brief period of time. Her experience of both mother and aunt was quite negative and rejecting. This rejection was due to her mother's numerous men friends and her aunt's complete devotion to her church. Her mother had many men friends, some of whom lived with her, others who she dated. In contrast, her aunt was totally devoted to the church, not only going to services on Sunday but also going to mass daily, often insisting that Rachel accompany her.

After some early satisfaction in the beginning process of studying to become a nun at her aunt's encouragement, her interest began to wane. She then decided she wanted to become a nurse and began studying for a degree in nursing.

While Rachel's perimenopausal state was never mentioned until the conclusion of our work together, looking back, the unconscious was clearly aware of this state, but it remained unknown to both of us. Please notice the abundance of the color, red, and some of the shapes that are created in her trays.

Figures 3.26-3.29 (Rachel Tray 1)

Her first tray was created with great enthusiasm. In the central position is a tyrannical masculine figure, who invades her inner and outer worlds. She said that the guy standing on the bridge was a devilish guy who uses his trident to bully people around. She described him as a slave driver.

I noted the passive mermaid just lounging on a rock in the background. I was pleased to see the trees, natural organic growth, as well as the cuddling couple in the right-hand corner. I saw these as hopeful signs of what was possible for her internally, as well as what she might be able to actualize in the outer world. These gave me hope that this process could move in a positive direction.

Early in our work, Rachel's relationship with a married man became the main topic of conversation. For over five years she had been in this relationship, and he constantly promised to leave his wife and marry her. He never did.

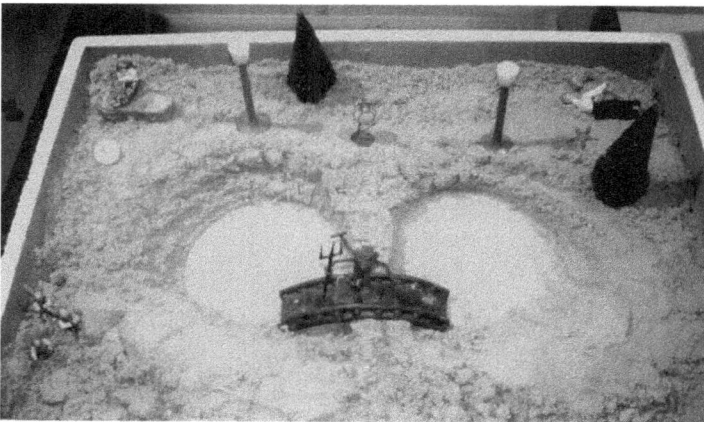

Figure 3.26 Rachel's Tray 1

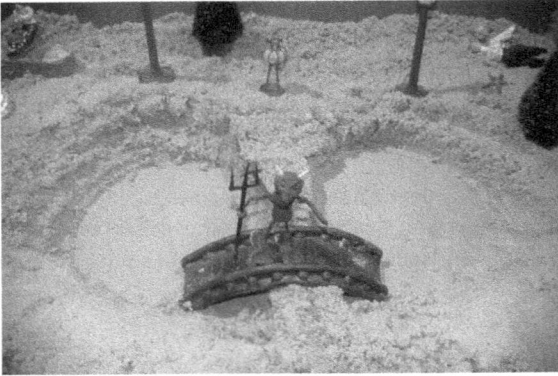

Figure 3.27 Rachel's Tray 1

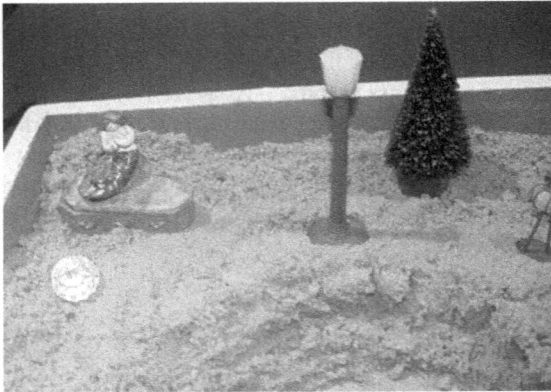

Figure 3.28 Rachel's Tray 1

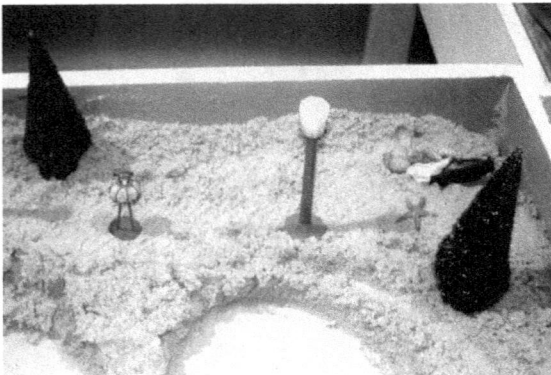

Figure 3.29 Rachel's Tray 1

Figure 3.30 - 3.33 (Tray 2)

About four months into therapy, Rachel took a long time shaping the sand in what looked to be a butterfly – much later I wondered if these were fallopian tubes. At the time, I wondered if she was giving shape to her own unfolding, emerging Self. Certainly something was in the process of transformation. Then, on top of this shape, where the split continues to be depicted, is once again the same old devil. Notice the barrier she now makes between the two sides. At the same time something quite astonishing is occurring. The devil that she used in the first tray is now facing Ganesha, the elephant-headed Hindu god.

Ganesha gets invoked at the beginning of a journey because he and only he has the power to remove obstacles and to place the person on the path to success. This Hindu god bears some striking similarities to Rachel's life journey. In one myth of Ganesha's early life, he

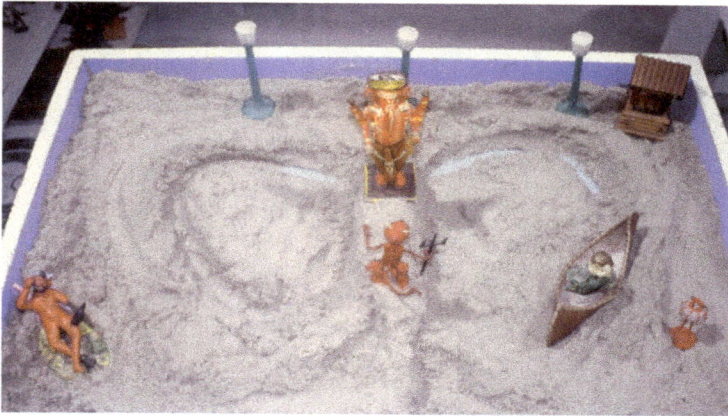

Figures 3.30 Rachel's Tray 2

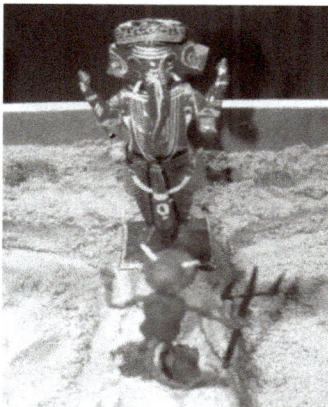

Figure 3.31 Rachel's Tray 2

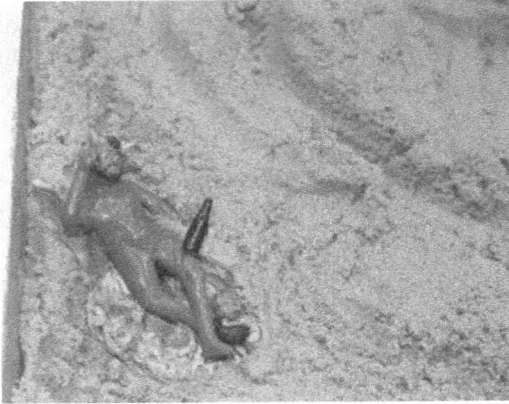

Figure 3.32 Rachel's Tray 2

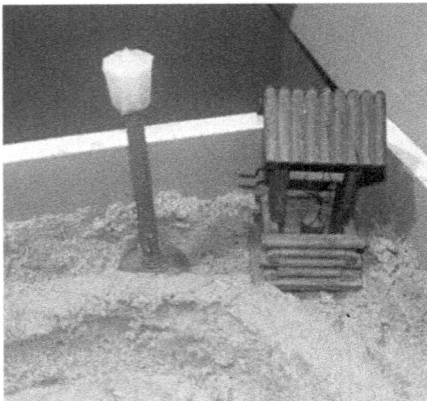

Figure 3.33 Rachel's Tray 2

was separated from his mother soon after birth. Eventually he was reborn into wholeness. In this tray, Ganesha faces the old tyrannical, patriarchal attitudes (symbolized by the devil) that have been in power up until now. Perhaps, now, this confrontation will now allow Rachel's own feminine nature to emerge.

Rachel said, "I like the wishing well the very best in the tray." Now she is able to connect to this well, which just might connect her to the waters of her deepest self.

Figures 3.34 - 3.36 (Tray 3)

The split continues but now in the shape of a butterfly. Her energy is clearly moving toward a more defined, organized, and unified Self than ever before. Her own fire has been ignited in the images of the red hands and red hearts, now more unified and more together here than

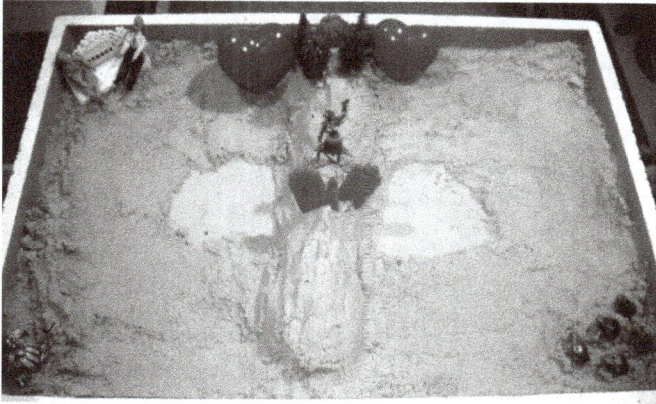

Figure 3.34 Rachel's Tray 3

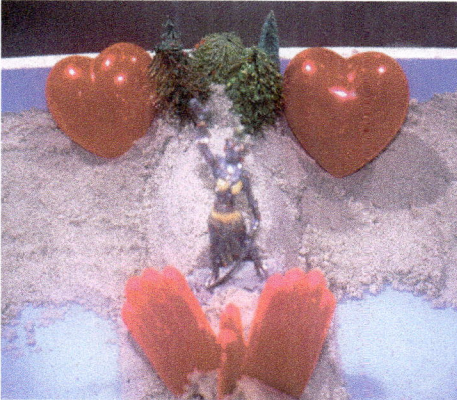

Figure 3.35 Rachel's Tray 3

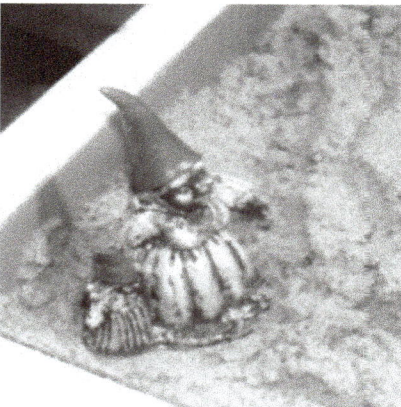

Figure 3.36 Rachel's Tray 3

ever before, taking center stage, and unifying the two sides of herself. Now her own natural fire and energy, in the form of the two red hands and two red hearts, is in a central position. Her blood is freely flowing now, and that is what burns and lights up the scene. Looking back on her work, I see more in the fire than I did then. I also wondered if this fire could have been referring to the heat of hot flashes. At this point, she was in her mid-forties.

Hidden behind the bush is a strong and vital woman, a woman who is able to take up the sword herself. I hoped that this woman was a depiction of Rachel's increasingly strengthened ego. The mother and child in the front corner are perhaps a continuing statement to me about her transference feelings.

Not long after she made this tray, she stopped the relationship with her married lover. For the first time, she was able to keep her promise to herself that she would have absolutely no contact with him. And she didn't.

Figures 3.37 - 3.39 (Tray 4)

As Rachel worked on this picture, she continued to feel uncertain about whether she should show me the figure she put behind the fences, the figure that is in front of the fire and is hidden. Here we see her reluctance to reveal her feminine essence – of such central importance. She is hiding an ancient pregnant woman, an eternal image of rebirth and regeneration throughout the ages. I believe her ambivalence was about showing this much of this side of her Self.

In this tray her real feelings and drives are emerging, symbolized by the natural fertile mound, the trees, the water in the pond, the two bridges, and the pregnant goddess hidden from front view. The single mother and child continue to overlook the situation, now from an even better perspective.

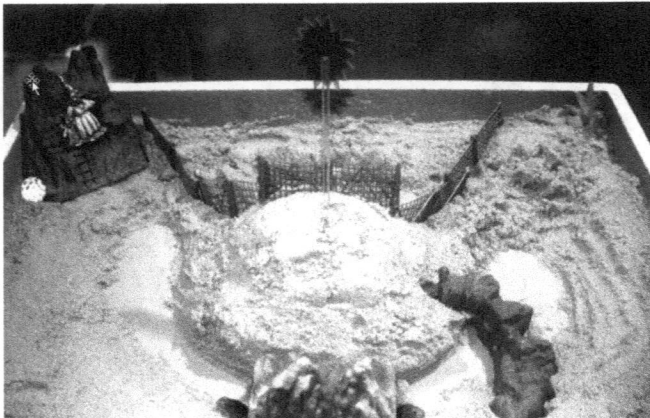

Figure 3.37 Rachel's Tray 4

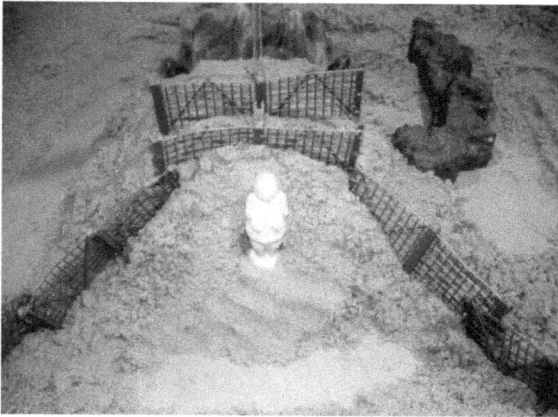

Figure 3.38 Rachel's Tray 4

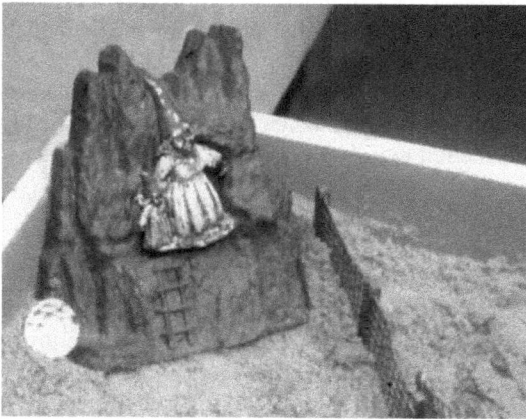

Figure 3.39 Rachel's Tray 4

Figure 3.40 (Tray 5)

For the first time, Rachel created only one central circular space in the sand, upon which she placed a skeleton. In front of the skeleton, she put two gravestones, each on a mirror, with one fiery red hand in front of the gravestones. Behind the skeleton, she placed three gold shells. All the miniatures in the tray are behind this hand, as though this activity is being blessed. She placed fire in the four corners. Rachel's only comment about this particular tray was "the fires on the outside will eventually burn up this death scene."

At the time, I wondered what was getting ready to be burned and destroyed. Was the skeleton a depiction of the end of her fruit-bearing years? I also wondered, as she made the circle

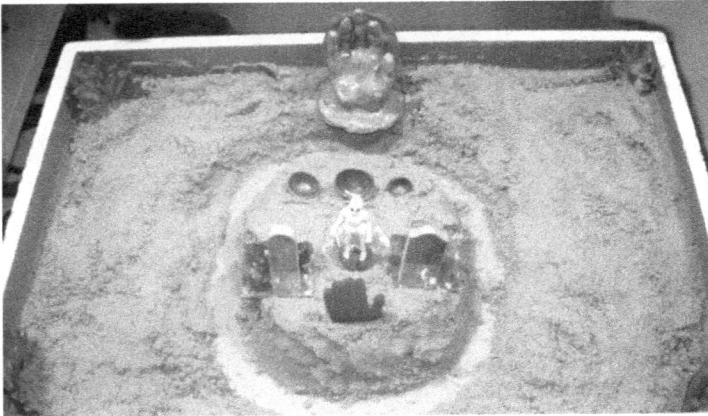

Figure 3.40 Rachel's Tray 5

in the sand, if she was participating in a ritual marking the new phase of her womanhood. As she filled the four corners with fire, I noted that she had much psychic energy that seemed to move her on. It was as though she was "cooking" on the inside. Were these the fires of change that were burning or perhaps more indications of hot flashes?

In outer life, Rachel was beginning to actualize the new direction. She now had moved into psychiatric nursing in another city and recently had taken a meaningful internship at a small local hospital for women. She said she felt ready now for whatever came her way with this big move.

Figure 3.41 (Tray 6)

Rachel created this tray slowly and with much care. She said, "I loved making this shape and the feel of putting my hands right smack into the center. I've never made this much room for myself in the sand before – ever." This tray suggests that her center, the Self, is becoming more consolidated and less fragmented and split, making her life energy more available.

About three months after she had begun her hospital internship, she met a man while working in the hospital. They enjoyed each other's company and began spending time together. He was not Catholic but from a religion of which her aunt violently disapproved. She was both happy about being with him but also troubled about the vast religious and age differences.

Three months later, she created this tray, working hard to create the central solid mountain. It took her almost the entire session to finish the tray, enveloped in silent concentration throughout. It was only at the last moment that she put the fiery red hand on top of the mountain. When I saw this symbol, I reviewed in my mind her various uses of fire – sometimes to cleanse, sometimes defensively, sometimes to reaffirm her own energy, and now as a marker of her achievement.

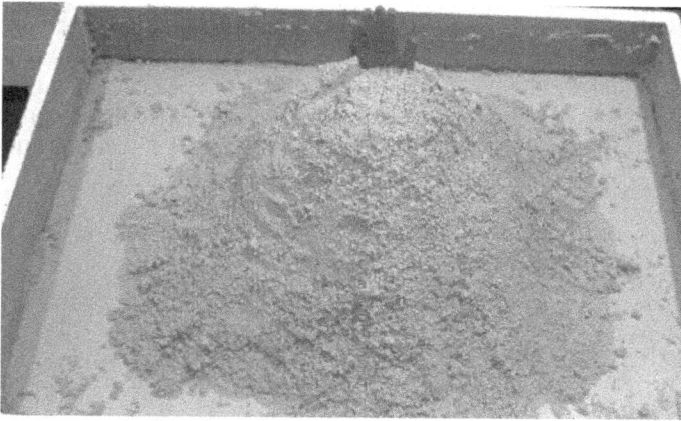

Figure 3.41 Rachel's Tray 6

It wasn't long after creating this tray that she and her male friend decided to get married. She said that she felt ready to deal with whatever came up as a result of that decision.

Figure 3.42 (Tray 7)

Once again Rachel energetically created a large circular mound in the center, this time crowned by a flower that she went into my garden to pick, a natural element symbolizing her own natural center and a direct connection of her transference feelings for me. This tray was a solid depiction of the consolidation of the Self in relation to the ego and centered enough to help her proceed on her way.

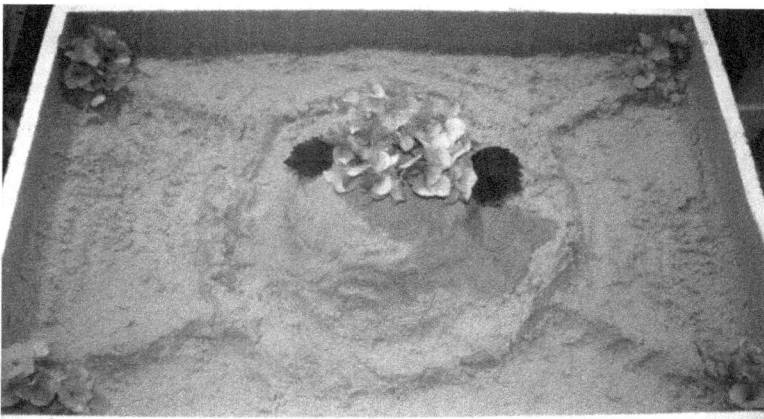

Figure 3.42 Rachel's Tray 7

Figure 3.43 (Tray 8)

This tray was created one month after her wedding. She told me that this was a center with two moons. Ancient as well as current wisdom recognizes a woman's nature as cyclical, like the moon and the tides. A woman's energy waxes, shines full, and then wanes again.

She told me that she was feeling more solid, settled, and less chaotic than ever before and that it felt like a miracle. My personal fantasies about what she was depicting in the tray were of two lovers spooned together or the transference and countertransference between us; perhaps it was also what she had never experienced as a child, the original mother-child unity.

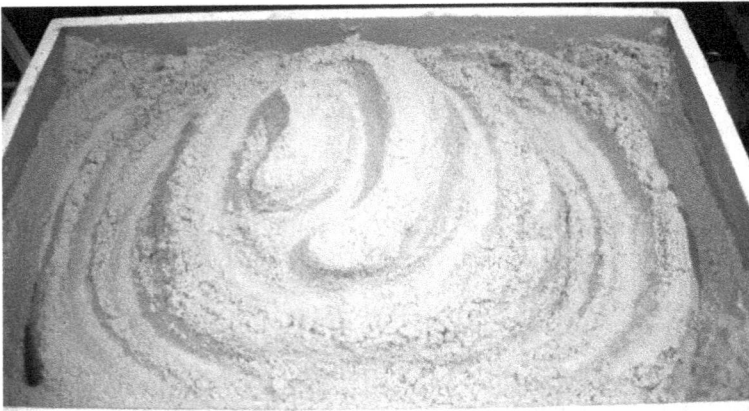

Figure 3.43 Rachel's Tray 8

Figure 3.44 (Tray 9)

Rachel had recently turned 50. She had also seen her gynecologist the week before, and the doctor had told her that it was clear from her lab tests that she was now menopausal. She was totally surprised by this news.

After she created this tray she said, "I have never felt myself coming together internally as I felt when I made this tray." She said, "I can see my uterus and vagina in a totally new and much clearer way. It's funny, even though I'm moving into menopause, it looks as though there's a birth canal as well as something that's ready and willing to receive it."

I believe that she had birthed her creative feminine self; this was a true psychological birthing and at this moment she was feeling the fullness of psychological birth.

She also told me that her husband finds her sexually attractive, a real turn on, and this pleased her enormously. A vital connection and new sense of aliveness had occurred within her body, spirit, ego, and innermost Self in a most dramatic way, and she was living it fully.

In the containment of our protected space, sandplay had become an important means by which Rachel could let herself be guided by the internal wisdom of the archetypal psyche.

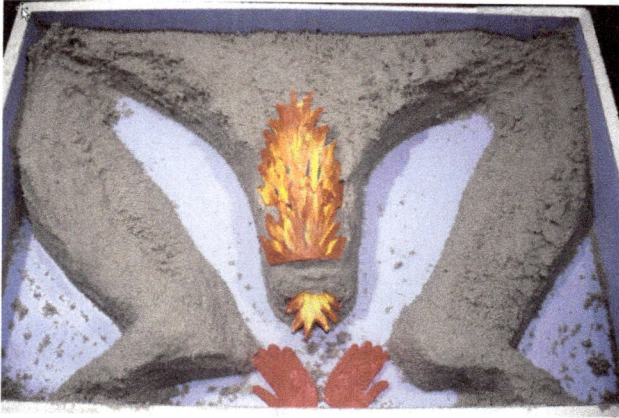

Figure 3.44 Rachel's Tray 9

This connection had led her into her own feminine mystery and had initiated her into this new transition. Rachel was now living a much fuller and more satisfying life.

In closing

All of these women had been able to use their therapeutic work, enhanced by the sandplay experience, to contact the archetypal depths of their psychic life and to find initiation rites that would move them on in their personal lives.

References

Bradway, K. (c. 1980). Personal communication to H. S. Friedman.

Jung, C.G. (1967a). *The collected works of C.G. Jung: Symbols of transformation* (Vol. 5, p. 190). Princeton University. (Original work published 1960).

Jung, C.G. (1967b). *The collected works of C.G. Jung: Two essays on analytical psychology* (Vol. 7, p.114). Princeton University. (Original work published 1960).

Jung, C.G. (1971). *The collected works of C.G. Jung: Psychological types* (Vol. 6, p.66). Princeton University. (Original work published 1921).

Neumann, E. (1973). *Quoted in Journeys, Encounters: Clinical, Communal, Cultural: Proceedings of the 17th Congress of the International Association for Analytical Psychology* (pp.167, 186). Cape Town 2007.

Chapter 4

Childhood loss

Losing a parent or experiencing a different traumatic experience early in life has an enormous impact on a child. The impact is not only immediate; it can also change how the child sees his/her life, as well as how the child's entire life is lived. Sandplay helps these children (as well as adults) express and understand the effects of early horrific life experiences and thus helps them repair the damage.

Jungian trauma work, attachment theory, and/or neuroscience research can provide useful information about how the psyche repairs itself, as well as how the young brain develops and the best conditions under which a child can grow and learn.

For example, the nonverbal technique of sandplay therapy bypasses the thinking process and activates the internal wisdom of the body, as well as the deep internal wisdom of the unconscious. Deep in the unconscious there is a natural tendency, given the proper conditions, for the psyche to heal itself with the help of internal images. Just as our physical wounds heal under certain conditions, the psyche also has the instinctual wisdom to heal itself if it is left free to operate naturally in a protected and safe environment. The nonverbal technique of sandplay helps activate this profound level of the psyche and helps the psyche to heal.

This chapter begins with an overview of the effect and extent of traumatic experiences. Then, it discusses how loss is perceived from three perspectives: Jungian theory, attachment theory, and neuroscience research. Finally, excerpts from several child and adult sandplay cases are discussed. The cases deal with the experience of loss and then movement toward healing.

There are many ways that an experience of loss can affect children. For example, loss can severely impact normal development, especially if it occurs at an early age. Or, to avoid memory of painful early traumas, necessary defenses are sometimes erected into the psychic system, which may interfere with further growth.

What is trauma? Trauma is an event in which a person witnesses or experiences a threat to his/her own life or physical safety or the lives and physical safety of others and the experience of fear, terror, and/or helplessness that accompanies such a threat. Trauma is an intense and almost unbearable emotional experience brought about by such events as abuse, loss of a parent, divorce, or some other assault to one's sense of safety. Traumatic events challenge an individual's view of the world as a just, safe, and predictable place. It is our job as therapists to help clients contain and understand these fears and the accompanying psychic pain. Donald Kalsched (1997, 2013) maintains that when trauma happens in an early pre-verbal time in life – before the ego has developed and the normal defenses have had time to develop and protect the personality – it feels to the child like an emotional catastrophe.

Surveys on loss have found that many children who have had traumatic experiences could have been helped by receiving psychological treatment. The data also reveal that many children do not have treatment. Five percent of all children under 15 lose a parent to death. In the United States, 50% of all urban inner-city youth under the age of 20 have experienced the sudden and unexpected death of a close relative or friend (These statistics are not related to war or natural disasters). The research on loss and trauma indicate that these issues become part of individuals' life-long patterns and predispose them to (a) feelings of unmet longing, (b) fear of separation, (c) masked or unmasked depression, (d) hopelessness and feelings of being alone, and (e) continued feelings of father and/or mother hunger throughout their lives (Wallerstein, 2000).

One important research study (Wallerstein, 2000, p.xxxiii–xxxvi) found that the risk of depression escalates for children and adults who have suffered the loss of a parent in childhood. Eighty percent of all adults who suffer chronic depression were found to have lost a parent before they were 15 years old. Only half of these adults were found to cope and successfully adapt. The other half reported that they had never felt they had adapted adequately to their life circumstances, even decades later. In another study of children who had lost a parent (Wallerstein, 2000, p.294–301), it was demonstrated that "the unconscious, as well as the conscious sensitivity of these children can be 50 times more acute than that of a normal child." A loss of a parent feels like an amputation of a limb and results in feelings of helplessness and depression. Children learn early on to be wary and to defend against any further loss and feelings of high anxiety.

An interesting study) conducted on early parent loss and mental illness (Wallerstein, 2000, p.26–38) indicated that it was not just the early parent loss that predisposed a child to subsequent mental illness; it was the quality of the caretaker's replacement that was the crucial factor in the child's future mental health. The circumstances and people that surround a child after the death of a parent appear to have a profound effect upon the child's mental health. However, additional important factors also need to be considered when determining the effects of loss on an individual, including the age and life circumstances of the child or adult when the loss was experienced.

Divorce is another type of traumatic event for all the family members, especially the children. The trauma may occur at the time of the parents' separation or the trauma may continue well into adulthood, depending on the circumstances that follow. For example, additional traumatic feelings may be created if the divorce is one where the conflict continues after the separation and is ongoing between the parents causing continued confusion and anxiety.

Change in the family through divorce can have an enormous impact on a child. In the United States, 40% or more children have witnessed the breakup of their parents' marriage before they reach the age of 18. For children who have divorced parents, the divorce may determine how they see their world in the future and may also affect relationships with others.

Judith Wallerstein, a researcher in the United States, conducted a long-term study examining the effects of parental divorce on children. In this research, 131 children whose parents separated when they were between the ages of 2 and 6 were studied for 25 years. Both the children and their parents were interviewed regularly over these many years. The most important findings were:

1. Half of the children, before the age of 14, were involved with drugs and alcohol
2. The girls were inclined to become sexually active as young adolescents

3. One-third of the children did not continue their education after high school and only a fairly low percentage of those who went to college actually graduated from college
4. One-quarter of the individuals, now in their 20s and early 30s, are married. Two of those young married couples have divorced already. Another quarter of the group did not date. The remaining young people seem to be more in search of causal, uncommitted relationships than long-lasting relationships (Wallerstein, 2000, 2003)

Recent studies suggest that divorce has a greater immediate effect on boys than on girls. Boys from divorced families show more aggressive and acting out behaviors and less social ability than boys in non-divorced families. Girls are just as likely to be troubled by marital turmoil as boys, but they tend to demonstrate their feelings by becoming anxious and withdrawn. In late adolescence and young adulthood, when their relationships move to center stage, their own relationships with the opposite sex are often very conflicted – they are frightened of being abandoned and betrayed. One of the long-term effects for women from divorced families is a very high divorce rate.

A different study done by Wallerstein (2000, p.14–25) found that 70% of children in psychotherapy were from divorced families. With regard to adolescents, she found that 80 to 100% of adolescents in inpatient mental health settings were from divorced families. The high percentages of children and adolescents in treatment inform us about the many children and adults whose lives have been profoundly affected by divorce.

Considerable evidence suggests that children from homes with inter-parental conflict, whether they are broken or intact homes, are at greater risk than are children from broken or intact homes that are relatively harmonious. Conflict between parents has been associated with behavior problems in children, whether that conflict occurred in intact marriages, before a divorce, or after a divorce. A major study of more than 20,000 children in Great Britain (Millennium Cohort Study, 2018) found that children whose parents are married but have long-standing intense conflict are worse off than children from divorced homes. Children in families wracked by intense conflict, violence, and substance abuse would be better off if their parents split up. However, in the average divorce, where one parent is merely bored or unfulfilled, children are not better off if parents divorce.

One of the major effects of marital discord and divorce on children is the loss of a figure who was closely attached, thereby producing fear and anxiety. Therefore, divorce involving separation from either parent has a direct negative effect on the child, and this is an important factor to consider. However, it is the ongoing conflict that causes an ongoing sense of confusion and an unsettled state of mind.

It is important to remember that, while traumatic experiences are initially negative, positive experiences coming from these changes may also help lead to new growth in a child or adult. We all are aware of children and adults, despite experiences of overwhelming loss, who go on to have fulfilling and productive lives and who are able to maintain long and loving relationships. It is important to understand that the psyche has a huge capacity to compensate for early wounding and to make a positive recovery from the many traumas that children endure.

Now, consider some findings from brain research (Siegel, 1999; Siegel and Bryson, 2012) about the shocking and powerful influence that loss and trauma have on the psyche and developing brain. During the first 18 months of life, when the brain is going through a huge growth spurt, personal attachment experiences profoundly affect the brain's development. Also, when trauma or loss is experienced in this early stage of development, the young brain is affected in a negative way because traumatic experiences affect the developing autonomic system in the brain and this leads to structural changes in the brain. These structural changes produce inappropriate coping behaviors, such as dissociation. For example, if a baby is allowed to remain too long in a frantic state of distress and experiences states of unbearable fear and terror, then dissociation may result. This pattern of dissociation as a defense mechanism in times of stress or anxiety is likely to continue throughout that individual's life.

Research using neuron-imaging techniques tells us that psychotherapy does indeed have the possibility of physically changing the brain and making new life changes possible. This research suggests that more brain centers and pathways in the brain get activated and are formed when people are involved in hands-on symbolic activity than any other form of communication. This information supports the use of sandplay for both children and adults who are able to express this earlier experience of unbearable loss in the presence of a caring witness.

Individuals who have had early traumatic experiences can, in therapy, access the deepest level of the psyche and find the healing energy there in order to connect to the positive life pull that can help them return to their own life issues. Through sandplay, clients can reclaim and connect to their own natural way of being and develop an ego to deal with their outer life issues. Sandplay helps clients fight off the pull toward the past and feelings of depression and emptiness. It is this positive inner shift toward life that is supported both by the therapy and sandplay.

From a Jungian perspective, when there is a damaged or lost relationship to the parents, a child becomes much more vulnerable to the destructive and frightening aspects of the unconscious; this is likely to activate negative and frightening images. Jungian theorists see early experiences with the parents and caregivers in childhood as activating primordial archetypes. They stress that it is the parents' role to help the child mediate and regulate these instinctual responses. The "good-enough" human experience is made possible through those parents and caregivers being personally caring, mirroring their children's experiences, and being involved with them. A damaged relationship with mother or father makes the child vulnerable to the more destructive and frightening aspects of the unconscious and activates a more negative side of the parental images (Siegel & Bryson, 2012; Kalsched, 2013).

How do these traumatic issues appear in sandplay creations

Figure 4.1

This four-and-a-half-year-old boy initially tried to put the figures into the tray standing up, but when he could not keep them standing up, he quickly dumped them all over the tray. This young boy's older brother had recently been injured in a car accident; he had been in the same car accident and he had not been hurt at all. This child was feeling responsible and guilty for this terrible accident. This tray was just like how he felt inside, with many feelings, most of them very confused (**Figure 4.1**).

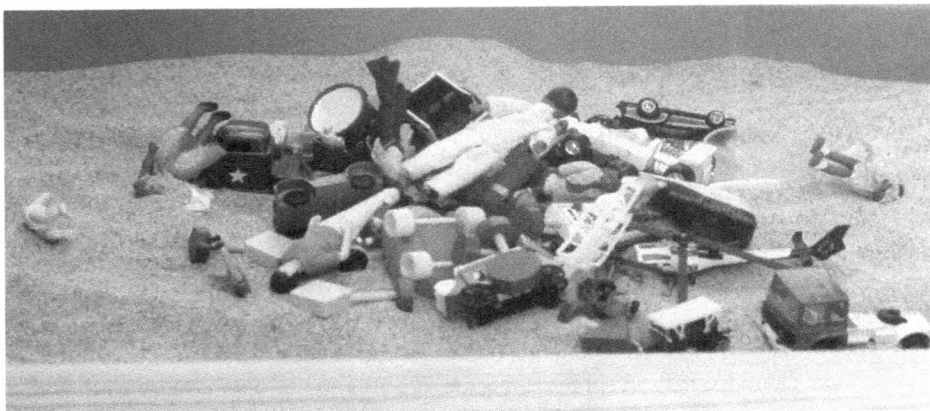

Figure 4.1 Tray of a four-and-a-half-year-old boy

Figure 4.2

When I looked at this five-year-old boy's sandplay, I thought of an infant, feeling over-whelmed but trying so hard to help himself. His parents had divorced a few months earlier, and his father had told his mother and this child that he was going to get married again. Mother was upset and crying a lot of the time. The boy felt lost with the sudden absence of support by either Mom or Dad. He had recently started bed-wetting again. He couldn't control that either, but the tray shows how hard he is trying. We see the repetitive lining up of various vehicles. Note the wedding couple in the tray in the middle of it all.

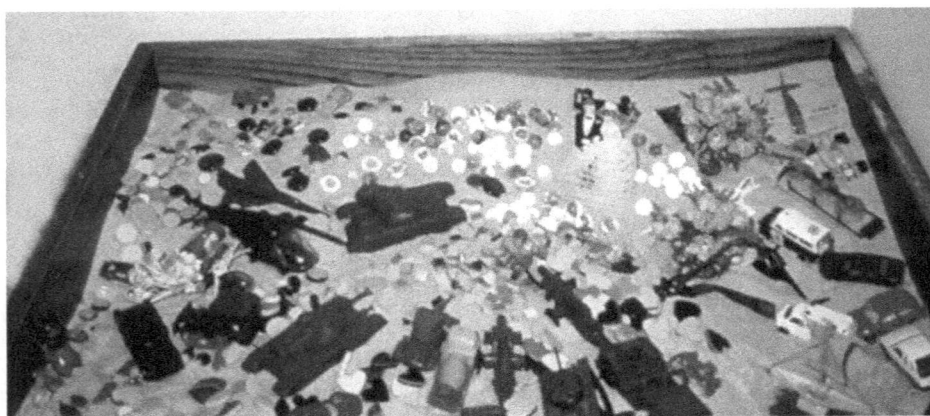

Figure 4.2 Tray of a five-year-old boy

Figure 4.3

This sandplay was created by a ten-year-old boy, whose father had just been taken to prison for embezzling money from his employer. His mother was full of feelings of rage, abandonment,

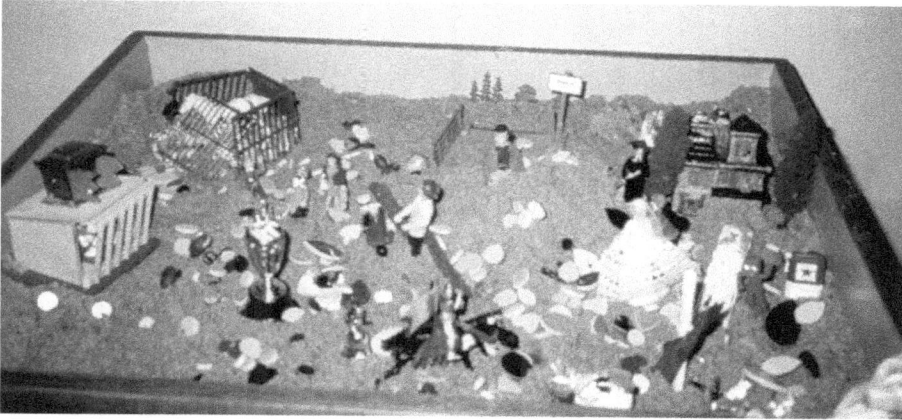

Figure 4.3 Tray of a ten-year-old boy

and great shame. This child is trying hard to contain himself. Notice how he tries to contain some of the chaos by building cages (perhaps prisons?) in which he was putting his feelings. This child is using the tray to express both his and mother's rage at the shame of the father's behavior and where it left them both.

Figure 4.4

This six-year-old girl's father had been murdered one year before this tray was created. Mother's ex-husband had shot him when they were all in an argument. The child had been in the next room. Now, a year later, this girl had become numb and withdrawn from the world. She was still trying to stop the terrible, frightening feelings inside her, what she had seen and

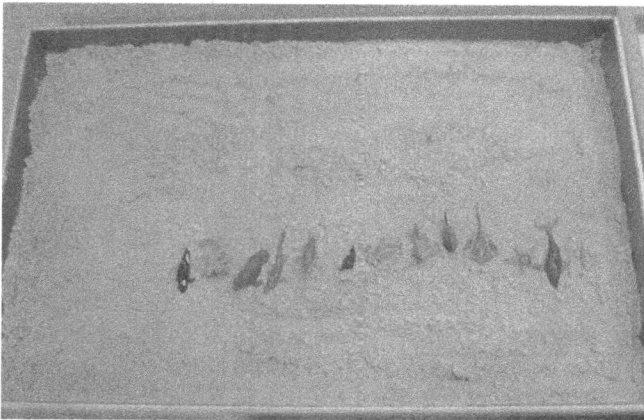

Figure 4.4 Tray of a six-year-old girl

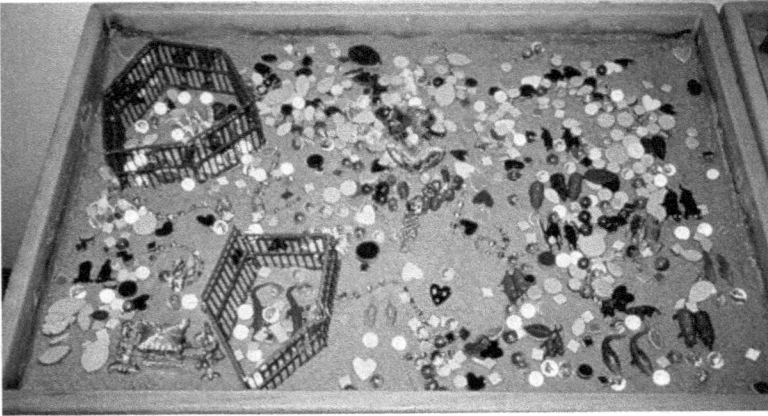

Figure 4.5 Tray of an eight-year-old girl

heard, as well as the loss of her father. During therapy, she said that she was very sad and didn't feel safe anywhere any more. She had been a lively child – now she was a silent and withdrawn child. She became such a "good and quiet girl" that it frightened her mother. This child had gone into psychological hiding – we can see how she lined up all these sea creatures – and fell into a very big depression at home and at school. This double trauma sent her into a place where she turned away from it all, trying to find a safe place.

Figure 4.5

This eight-year-old girl felt fearful and trapped between her divorced and angry parents. Father was very strict and controlling with her; mother was indulgent and over-protective. The mother also was fearful of confronting her ex-husband about the money that he gave her for support. This girl felt overwhelmed and confused by their arguments, fearful and angry with them both. She was brought to me on her teacher's suggestion, after she had begun taking things from other children at school. This scattered and disorganized tray reflected her innermost feelings and her attempt to develop a relationship with each of her parents, as represented by the two fenced off areas.

Case of Anna

To illustrate how the healing process unfolds in a clinical case, three selected sandplay scenes created by "Anna," a middle-aged woman, are discussed in light of various theoretical perspectives. Specifically, we consider: (a) parallels between her background and imagery in the sand; (b) Anna's willingness to participate in sandplay and how this influenced her trays; (c) her approach in creating a sand scene and what that suggested; (d) her first tray (based on Kalff and Friedman's observations on initial trays); (e) symbolic content and possible meanings; (f) her use of wounding and healing themes over time; (g) developmental guidelines; (h) Anna's comments and stories about her sandplay pictures; (i) therapist's feeling responses to the trays; and (j) transference issues. Rather than discussing each point separately, an overall view of Anna and her process is covered to provide a more organic understanding of Anna's work in the sand.

Background information

Anna was a married Caucasian woman with five grown children. When she began therapy, her youngest child was 17 and the only one living at home. She began therapy because of dissatisfaction with her life as a wife, mother, and secretary. She was experiencing stomach distress due to food allergies that limited her physical functioning and kept her from seeking a more satisfying job commensurate with her abilities and interests, as well as from expressing herself in her usual creative way through art.

Initially, her considerable intelligence was not apparent to me, as she appeared to be fragile, insecure, and blocked in expressing her thoughts and feelings. She seemed to be in physical pain much of the time. As I began to know her better, I felt that the pain was an underlying symptom of her emotional distress rather than its cause.

As the work proceeded, I increasingly came to realize that Anna was a bright, insightful, and imaginative woman who had suffered from a background of repression. The fundamentalist religious environment in which she had grown up supported her natural artistic talents only to a point, valuing them only to the degree that they could contribute to the church and to her own home later, as a mother. Her parents supported this narrow viewpoint by not allowing her to pursue interests in music and art when she entered a religiously affiliated college. She obediently majored in homemaking. Growing up with a compliant nature in such a limiting environment created a lifetime pattern of repressed feelings and submissive responses.

Near the beginning of therapy, Anna hesitantly shared her uncertain memories of occasional sexual abuse by her step-grandfather when she was a visitor in his home from ages 10 to 14. Although she tried to push this out of her mind by telling herself that she was wrong – it hadn't really happened – memories continued to haunt her throughout her adolescence and into adulthood. She never spoke with her parents about the events or her feelings during these years, nor did she receive any recognition from them that something might have happened. Their lack of awareness, or possibly their refusal to acknowledge any untoward behavior, contributed to her feelings of self-doubt.

Anna selected me as her therapist because she knew, through another client, that I sometimes used sandplay and other nonverbal, creative techniques in working with children and adults. It was only a short time into treatment before it became clear that she was drawn to working in the sand. She clearly enjoyed this nonverbal modality and created 17 sand pictures during the first 11 months of therapy. Sometimes she made a scene every week; other times, one or two scenes a month. After the completion of the 17 scenes, Anna moved from the sand tray into an entirely verbal process for two years and nine months.

Three of Anna's sandplay scenes are presented here: her first tray, a middle tray, and the final tray (i.e., her 17th tray). These scenes provide a thumbnail sketch of how sandplay can help promote and activate a healing process within an ongoing, verbal therapeutic relationship. The sand trays also show how key issues are communicated through the pictures and how the scenes serve as a touchstone to indicate how Anna is progressing in treatment. In addition to sandplay, I used traditional verbal therapy with an eclectic mix of Rogerian client-centered therapy, Kohutian object relations theory, and Jungian-oriented dream work. At times, Anna was able to visualize symbols that arose spontaneously in her mind's eye and, when explored, related to her situation and offered further insight; therefore, this "Anna-originated" approach was used when the occasion presented itself.

Anna's first tray (Figure 4.6)

In creating this tray, Anna immediately descended into the deeper realm of the psyche and communicated important clues. In this way, I knew it was an initial tray rather than a super-ficial or persona tray. Her tray was a hopeful one, while also identifying painful issues. It communicated to me that she was open to using this modality to portray her inner struggles and that she had a strong connection to her unconscious with an easy ability to use symbols and play. The issues she presented were from long ago but were clearly alive now and were the source of her current distress.

When I first looked at her completed tray, I had two immediate responses: I felt over-whelmed and sad. I wondered if these feelings might be similar to Anna's feelings as well. Later I learned that these were, indeed, major feelings she was having about her life situation.

Anna's process in creating a tray began in a traditional manner. At my suggestion, she first touched the sand in the dry and wet trays, remarking that they both "felt good." With her hands resting palms-down in the wet sand, she slowly began to scan the miniatures. Suddenly her gaze seemed riveted, and she immediately reached for the ceramic flames (representing fire) located on a nearby shelf and quickly placed them in a double semicircle formation near the left corner of the wet tray. Pointing to the flames, Anna said, "This is energy, like a screen."

More slowly, Anna chose two additional miniatures: a leopard poised on a branch ready to strike and a wounded man on a stretcher carried by two medics. These she placed in the sand almost simultaneously: the leopard on a small ridge near the center, menacingly overlooking the wounded soldier and medics in the front of the tray. Next, a tombstone was placed in the right corner area and five hearts (one brown, three blue, and one pink) were positioned to cre-ate a semicircle in front of the stretcher. Last, Uhura, the communications officer from *Star Trek*, was placed behind the flames, separated from the other items in the tray. Anna identified

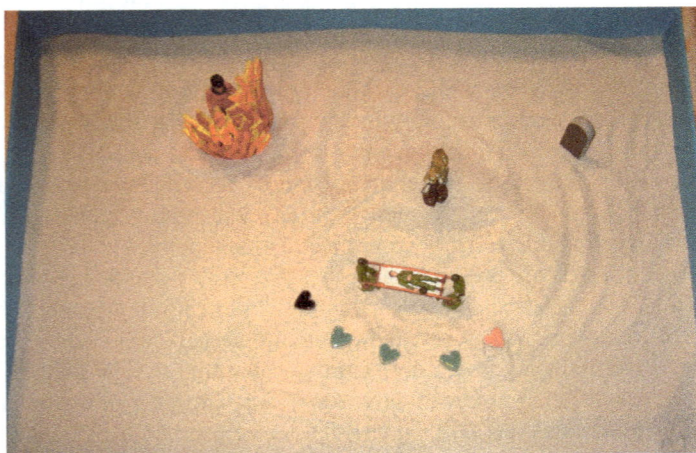

Figure 4.6 Anna's first tray

negative feelings were finally being expressed openly. Unconsciously, she is attempting to join these aspects, hoping to transcend her warring opposites (i.e., repressed feelings vs. consciously experienced ones) and unite them with a symbol of reconciliation (the bridge). I knew that if she were able to achieve this reconciliation, a new sense of self would transcend her divided state of self, as represented by the two mounds (Bradway, 1985). I could see how far she had come already, and I felt encouraged, for it seemed that she could trust our relationship enough to display these feelings.

In this tray, there are early indications of Anna's ability to bridge her many dark and destructive impulses and feelings. I was especially hopeful of Anna's use of the armadillo/dragon. The silent armadillo represents boundaries and the shield that protects humanity from all that is undesirable (Cooper, 1992). The fiery dragon is nearly the opposite symbol, a kind of amalgam of various animals that are particularly aggressive and dangerous, the primordial enemy with whom combat is the supreme test. According to Jung (1964), the dragon represents the shadow (i.e., the unconscious negative side of one's nature) that must be realized and integrated in the process of obtaining the treasures of inner knowledge and self-mastery. The armadillo/dragon figure Anna placed on the central bridge symbolizes a resourceful combination of both sets of attributes, dramatically illustrating her struggle, protective silence versus fiery rage. I wondered if now she might be closer to overcoming her fears and, eventually, to obtain the ultimate treasure.

In this tray, three themes of wounding are visible: splitting (e.g., the two mounds), hidden (e.g., the positioning of the heart, crocodile, and hippopotamus), and threatening (e.g., aggressive, powerful animals appearing so powerful that they might hinder new growth). Healing themes in the tray are: bridging (multiple bridges) and integrated (an organized scene encompassing the entire tray). Fewer wounding themes are contained in this tray than in Anna's initial tray, and the bridges suggest that she has already begun her healing journey to overcome her repressive patterns. While she still has much to confront, she is also exposing more than ever before. She is no longer hiding in the ground under the tombstone; now she is even partially exposed in the covered bridge. She will need the courage of the dragon and the protection of the armadillo to continue to encounter her repressed feelings and experiences.

Anna's final tray (Figure 4.8)

Six months after her ninth tray, Anna made her 17th and final sand picture. Energetically moving the sand, she created a central island and strategically placed a bridge that permitted full access to the "mainland." Included on the island is a large green tree growing out of a rock, a Bodhisattva, a swan, a mermaid, and a monkey. Water surrounds the island, and two rivers extend to the right side of the tray. The upper river goes in the direction of a newsstand shaded by trees next to an upright crystal. The lower river directly connects to two frogs sitting together on a lily pad, overlooked by a turtle. Nearby, a baby chick emerging from its shell lies within the protection of a seashell. This baby chick was the nearest miniature to where Anna was standing. On the far side of the tray, a sun rests on an elevated knoll, overlooking the entire scene. Nearby are a snake and two dead trees in contrast to the vibrant trees that she placed in the rest of the tray. In the lower left-hand corner, Anna carefully placed polished stones and jewels in front of another turtle.

My reaction to this tray was one of joy. From prior sandplay pictures, I knew that Anna's internal healing energies had been activated to aid her in dealing with her life issues. In this scene, the conflicts with which she had struggled for so long no longer took center stage. I

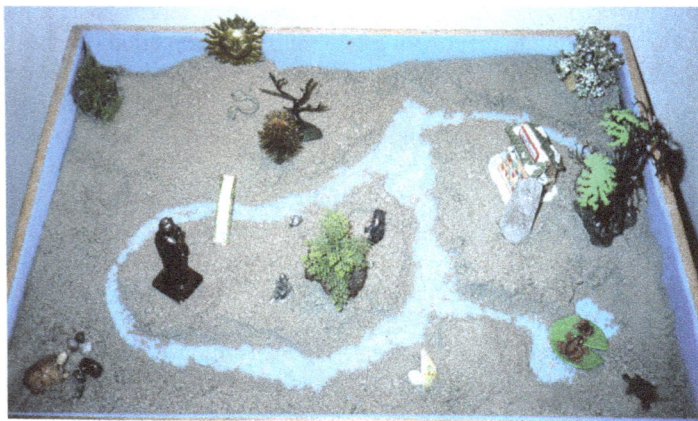

Figure 4.8 Anna's final tray

was struck by the organic nature of this scene – the imperfectly fashioned island, surrounded by water, with rivers gently reaching out to a world filled with trees, new life (baby chick), spiritual support (Bodhisattva), good health (monkey, credited in Asia with granting good health), and access to both land and water (i.e., the conscious and unconscious) through the mermaid, swan, frogs, and turtles. The sun, representing solar consciousness, was elevated, illuminating the entire scene. I wondered if her primitive rage, represented by the fire in her initial tray, had been transformed into a more conscious, mindful state where she now had the ability to overlook her world and to think objectively. The mermaid, Bodhisattva, and monkey appeared to be looking over the bridge, across the water, to the dead trees, snake, and sun. Was this another perspective bearing the reminder that difficult issues, in some form, are present in all of our lives? Or, might the bridge span the opposites as a symbol of reconciliation? Perhaps both?

When I saw the two frogs on the lily pad, I knew that Anna was feeling supported by me as she underwent her multiple changes. Her placement of the turtle nearby helped me understand that she, like the turtle, had been able to adapt and survive through decades of difficulties. When Anna completed the scene, she observed with amazement, "Here's an island – but it's connected! This is interesting – it isn't perfectly smoothed out. This (picture) feels fluid, life-like, offering options, movement." No longer does she have to be restricted to the achievement of perfection to please the old family and religious system that does not fit or support her creative nature.

Using the thematic approach in understanding Anna's trays helped me clarify and validate her process. In Anna's first and ninth scenes, the number of wounding themes far outnumber healing themes. In this final tray, no themes of wounding are present; there are only healing themes. A congruent, organized idea (i.e., her world) encompasses the entire tray (integrated) with an island in the center of the tray (centered theme). With the bridge joining the opposites (i.e., live tree/dead trees), a connection or reconciliation has occurred (bridging theme). The whole scene is alive with organic growth; vegetation is even growing out of a rock (energized theme). New development is emerging as the baby chick breaks out of its egg, so close where Anna is standing (birthing theme). The whole scene has a natural, spiritual quality that includes a Bodhisattva on the central island (spiritual theme). Now that these healing energies have been activated by this powerful process, I knew that they would continue to support her through her therapeutic experience – and, I hoped, throughout her life.

Reflection session

Six months after she created this final tray, Anna asked if I would be willing to review her trays with her. Although we were still immersed in verbal therapy, I agreed because I thought an objective look at her sandplay process would be helpful. Reflecting on her scenes was an enriching experience for both of us.

We then viewed all of her scenes. After she viewed her final tray, Anna looked visibly moved. She commented:

> It's like a celebration. This looks so eclectic, busy, hopeful, a lot of life – nowhere is it the same; it's unique. In the last tray, the swan feels really special to me. The turtle is carrying the treasure (the jewels) – like the specialness of who I am. I've discovered that I have a brain. The middle island is part of me, and it is connected to the whole of me. I'm such a different person now than how I was. I'm so much more whole. I'm accepting myself better, and I can rely enough on myself to spread out. I'm so much larger and have so many more options. Even if I'm afraid, I can spread out. I'm not alone. The whole tray is filled – a completion.

As I listened to her comments, it certainly seemed to me that the treasure had been found. By this later time, Anna's outer life mirrored her final sandplay scene. She had begun training as a massage therapist and enjoyed this work immensely. Later, after she had graduated and was about to open her own business, she quit her job as a secretary. She had begun to paint again. Her relationship with her husband felt easier and more satisfying; she experienced him as a more sensitive and empathetic partner with whom she was able to share and reflect on her feelings. No longer was she given to fits of rage in trying to communicate her frustration. Her allergic symptoms had lessened significantly with the help of a medical specialist.

Sandplay was an excellent technique to use with Anna. It tapped into her natural creative ability and allowed her to express, work through, and use her sharp mind to understand what had happened to derail her so early in life and cause such wounding. Anna's sandplay process was one of communicating, getting in touch with, understanding, and eventually integrating her negative and destructive emotions. She worked hard throughout therapy to repair the early rifts and understand her angry feelings, eventually gaining a new awareness of herself, becoming more comfortable with her body, and giving expression to her creative self.

Some final comments

Losses early in life have enormous impact on a child. The impact is not only immediate but can also persist throughout the individual's entire lifetime. Sandplay can help these children and adults to express and understand the effects of their early horrific life experiences. The self-healing properties of the psyche activated by sandplay can help repair the damage – in both children and adults.

References

Bradway, K. (1985). *Sandplay bridges and the transcendent function*. C. G. Jung Institute, San Francisco.

Cirlot, J.E. (1962). *A dictionary of symbols*. Philosophical Library.

Cooper, J. C. (1992). *An illustrated encyclopaedia of traditional symbols*. Thames & Hudson.

Jung, C. G. (1964). *Man and his symbols*. Doubleday.

Kalsched, D. (1997). *The inner world of trauma: Archetypal defenses of the spirit*. Routledge.

Kalsched, D. (2013). *Trauma and the soul: A psycho-spiritual approach to human development and its interruption*. Routledge.

Siegel, D.J. (1999). *The developing mind: How relationships and the brain interact to shape who we are*. Guilford Press.

Siegel, D.J., & Bryson, T.P. (2012). *The whole-brain child: 12 revolutionary strategies to nurture your child's developing mind*. Random House.

University College London Centre for Longitudinal Studies (2018). *Millennium cohort study*. https://cls.ucl.ac.uk/cls-studies/millennium-cohort-study/

Wallerstein, J. (2000). *Unexpected legacy of divorce; The 25-year landmark study*. Hyperion.

Wallerstein, J. (2003). *What about the kids?: Raising your children before, during, and after divorce*. Hachette Books.

Chapter 5

Recovering from childhood trauma

Jung emphasized the importance of transition rites for primitive cultures in moments of death. Historically, such experiences were mediated collectively in a holy place; Greeks called that holy space a *temenos*. Our modern culture offers us few rites of passage; the initiation necessary for psychological growth now happens through an individual crisis or a personal, life-changing event.

Joseph Campbell said: "Apparently, there is something in these initiatory images so necessary to the psyche that if they are not supplied from without, through myth and ritual, they will have to be announced again ... from within" (2004, p.7). These announcements frequently arise within the safe and protected *temenos* of the sandplay experience, as we who work with sandplay know so well.

Sandplay became the rite of passage for Margarita, a client in her early forties who suffered from emotional and physical trauma in her childhood. Sandplay provided the sacred container for her spontaneous initiation process to emerge. With the combination of the sand, a free and protected space, and the presence of an elder, an authentic experience emerged – uniquely personal, yet archetypal. The deep archetypal wisdom of the psyche constellated a rite of passage for her that filled the gap between modern society and ancient rites that were so necessary for developing the soul.

Her work showed the emergence and development of a creative, healing urge in the unconscious, and illustrates her personal journey with unusual purity and clarity. Margarita used a variety of materials to express the deep wounding she had to "suffer through" as she searched for a more meaningful way of life. One of the surprises of her inner work was the discovery of her creativity and the birth of her own inner artist.

Margarita grew up in a large family in what she called a *barrio*. She was the youngest of seven children. Her primary bond was with her father, with whom she felt the strongest sense of connection. Early on, she showed a vivid imagination and creative abilities, which her father, who also had a creative side, helped develop and encourage. They especially enjoyed painting and drawing together. Her relationship with her mother, however, was cold and distant, and she was not close to any of her siblings. Her teachers at school also recognized and encouraged her creative gifts. Margarita was a good student and did better at school than any of her sisters and brothers. As one would expect, these natural gifts, coupled with the attention from her father, brought on intense feelings of envy from both siblings and her mother.

Margarita adapted to her mother's and older sisters' envy by playing a Cinderella role – in other words, she survived as the youngest child in the family system by serving their needs and not her own. She became one of those children who early on stops listening to his/her own inner needs, hungers, and desires and instead becomes increasingly vigilant to the needs of his/her caretakers. It all seemed to work for her well enough until she was nine, when her father died suddenly of a heart attack. For Margarita, her father's death was an emotional catastrophe, a frightening abandonment. Her total capacity for an authentic relationship had been invested in him. Her caretaking adaptation worked well enough in the family when he was alive, but after his death, something in her died. At 13, Margarita's grandmother, with whom she shared some closeness, also died. At 15, two of her brothers were killed in a gang shoot-out.

Not surprisingly, the years following these accumulated losses were accompanied by profound depression. Her family and teachers did not recognize her depression but instead labeled her as a "daydreamer." By the time she finished high school, her self-esteem had diminished to a painfully low level. After high school, she decided to "take the plunge" and enter a Catholic order to become a nun. She didn't realize it at the time, but she was trying to give meaning to her life by choosing to turn to the church for containment and meaning, as her family had. The problem was that, throughout her training period to become a nun, she was plagued by feelings of emptiness, meaninglessness, and disappointment. Just before taking her final vows, Margarita began experiencing intense doubts, aware of the life-long commitment she was about to embrace. She felt panicky. She was so alarmed by these feelings that she abruptly left the convent. One night she packed up her things, drove off, and never returned.

Her departure from the Order brought on even greater feelings of despair. She had turned in hope toward another family, the church, but, like her personal family, she felt the church was not interested in listening to her needs, only insisting that she devote her life to serving others and bypassing herself. After this sudden leave-taking, she eventually drifted into a middle level government job as a secretary. At this point, in all aspects of her life, the avenues to her creative and imaginative nature were at a dead end. Her friendships were few as well. It was her natural introversion and love for reading that years later eventually led her to the more introspective writings of Thomas Merton. Then, through a circuitous route, she found her way to my office when she was in her early forties.

At the beginning of her therapy work, it was obvious that she was caught in a rigid role of serving her demanding and controlling family and upholding their traditional values and life style. Specifically, this included babysitting numerous nieces and nephews, caring for her aged and tyrannical mother, and volunteering at the church. She resented most of these chores. She ended up with little time for her own interests. This lifestyle made it difficult for her to connect to her own needs, to her own rich creativity, or even to her Mexican-American heritage.

By the time our work began, Margarita had come to see herself as a weak, passive woman only capable of leading a half-life; her "fire" had been essentially extinguished. Fewer and fewer personal choices seemed possible. In her early years, her natural impulses had been conditioned out of her by growing up in her home, attending parochial school, and serving the needs of the church.

Margarita's innate creativity had occasionally surfaced from time to time through the years. Periodically she tried painting or weaving, but with no support for her efforts she became easily discouraged and dropped them. But it was this creative thread, now supported by the therapy, where she able to bring her dreams and express herself in sandplay, that eventually facilitated her unique style.

In therapy there were many difficult and dark times for both of us. She was moody, she was silent, she couldn't find words with which to articulate her life experiences. Her profound

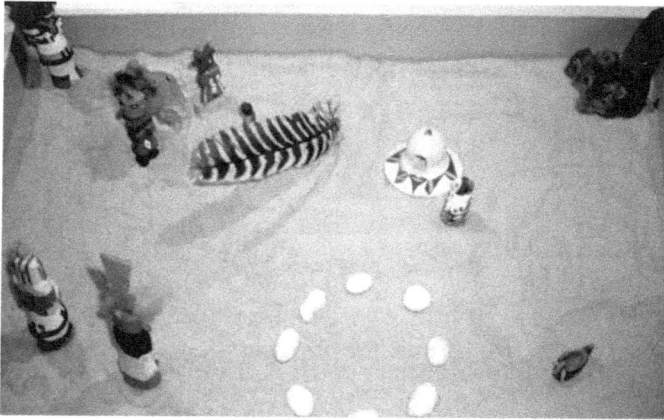

Figure 5.3 Tray 2

somewhere inside her. I wondered and hoped for just such a stable place. She placed a tiny empty canoe on the dry sand in the lower right corner, directionless and stuck. I was pleased to see the old masculine figure behind her in the upper right corner, suggesting that some separation from her dark past was beginning to take place. On the left side of the tray, she placed five Kachinas and a feather, protecting a small child.

Figure 5.4 (Tray 3)

Now, an old white male is placed off to the side, representing an alien system. In the clearing, shaped like a heart and connected to the bridge, is a glass bottle with a pearl encased inside. In Christianity it would be the "pearl of great price" – to be seen but still locked away and

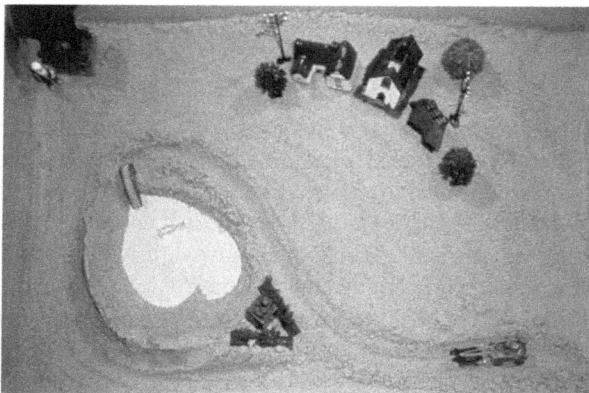

Figure 5.4 Tray 3

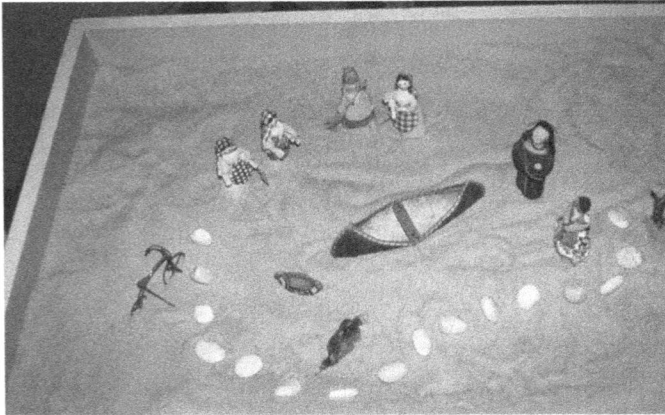

Figure 5.5 Tray 4

unattainable in the glass bottle. I hoped the pearl indicated that a treasure will emerge from dealing with her dark and painful material. The Buddha is close by. In the upper right is real life, still some distance away from the center. Even though distant, I was pleased to see it here. The telephone poles indicate the possible beginning of communication – certainly it had begun with me in our sessions at this point but also with this central place within herself. With the church so central, I wondered if perhaps she was trying to incorporate her earlier religious experience into her current outer life.

Figure 5.5 (Tray 4)

A large beached canoe is placed centrally, with a small canoe perpendicular to it. Both seem unable to move. Nearby is a small green animal. All are enclosed within the white shells and the observing women. A red bicycle is outside the circle.

Figures 5.6 – 5.8 (Tray 5)

Now, a most unusual event and unusual sandplay followed. Margarita phoned me ahead of our session to let me know that this day was the anniversary of her father's death and that she wanted to create a sand tray. She had never made a request like that before, announced her desire to talk about anything, or expressed a need to create a tray.

It was also unusual for Margarita to talk about her trays. After she had completed this tray and viewed it in silence for a long time, she said, "This is the graveyard with my dad, my brothers, and my grandmother. Now they've finally all come together."

In this scene, Margarita confronted and named the losses in her life. The losses occupy a central position, but they are also more contained and ready to be buried. The seed of her potential is here and set free at last, once her losses are consciously experienced and expressed. Four shells serve as gravestone markers. The overturned sundial shell was another

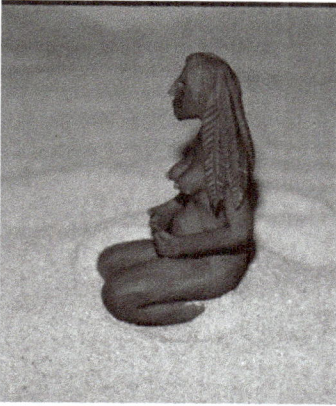

Figure 5.17 Margarita's 31ˢᵗ figure

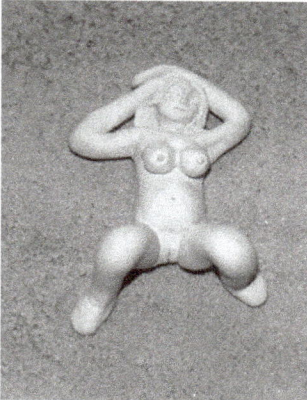

Figure 5.18 Margarita's 32ⁿᵈ figure

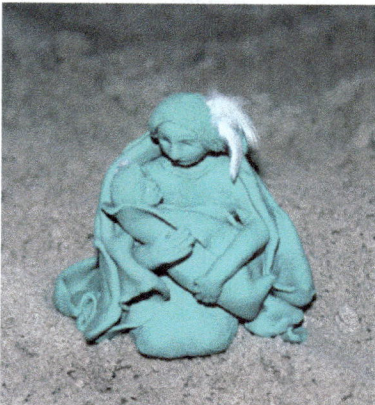

Figure 5.19 Margarita's 33ʳᵈ figure

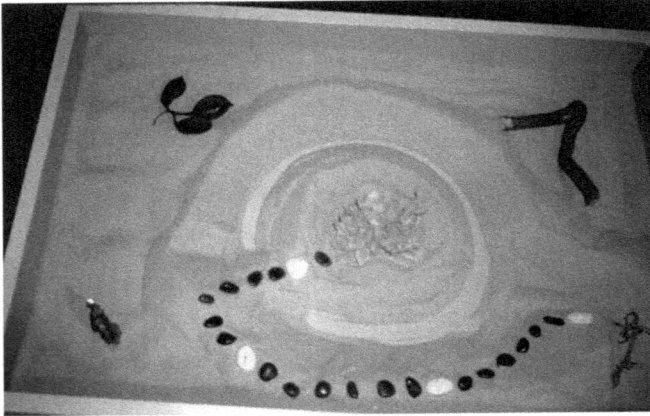

Figure 5.20 Margarita's Tray 7

as the vast spectrum of colors she used, indicated that she, herself, had gone through a "cooking" process. By the time this series of figures was completed, her depression had lifted, her old defenses and rigid attitudes both at work and at home had loosened, and she was getting along more easily with her co-workers and her family.

I was also impressed by the concrete changes she manifested in the outer world: she obtained two credit cards, arranged a loan from the credit union to build a new room in her house, and applied for a pay raise for which she had been eligible for some time. She was beginning to move out of her turtle shell to create a full life for herself.

Margarita created only three more sandplays after these sculpted objects stopped – and the objects stopped as suddenly as they began.

Figure 5.20 (Tray 7)

Here we see a clearer path, still winding, that leads to her own feminine center marked by a pink piece of coral, an open and vulnerable center, indicating how deeply she has been penetrated and also her new openness to life. Her path is clearly indicated by the integration of the black and white stones.

Figure 5.21 (Tray 8)

Finally, at last, she was able to focus on herself. In the center is a mirror that she carefully swept with the tiny broom. She had a place for herself in her own life now. I believe this sand tray shows her feeling of having truly been seen on her journey. It also comments on her new ability to self-reflect and see more than the sadness and abandonment of her early years, overseen by a woman of her own heritage.

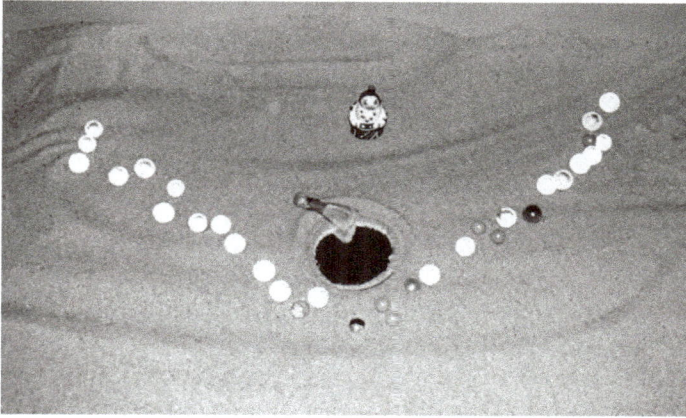

Figure 5.21 Tray 8

Figure 5.22 (Tray 9)

This final tray reminds me of an American Indian sand painting in the earth, now her own earth. I see the central image as representing the transformed masculine spirit. The circle that surrounds the sand painting is the *Zia*, or the sacred circle of protection. It provides absolute protection, as it is blessed by the central figure, a priest who invokes the protection from the gods themselves. I believe Margarita had felt protected in the therapy and, on some deep level, experienced our sessions, as well as the sandplay scenes, as sacred, protected by the gods themselves. This, to me, expressed Margarita's natural reverence and capacity for healing with these inner resources.

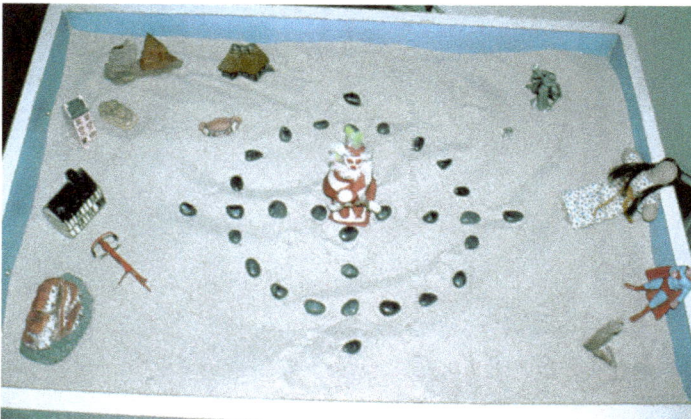

Figure 5.22 Tray 9

In the subsequent years, Margarita left her job and relocated to the Southwest United States, where she had felt drawn for a long time. In a recent phone conversation, she told me that her life is currently centered on her artistic pursuits, which continue to lead her into a life as an artist. She has received modest recognition from her community. I had the clear impression that she feels more seen, more heard, in this new life and that a genuine renewal has taken place.

References

Campbell, J. (2004). *The hero with a thousand faces* (3rd ed.). Princeton University Press. (Originally published 1949).

Kalff, D. (2003). *Sandplay: A psychotherapeutic approach to the psyche*. Temonos Press. (Originally published in English, 1980, by Sigo Press).

Chapter 6

Stages along the sandplay journey

Very early in her work, Dora Kalff observed that the symbolic imagery used in sandplay is related to the client's stage of ego development, as described by Neumann (1990, p.139). Kalff (1980) developed her developmental model along the same principles but adapted the stages for use in sandplay therapy. Her model simplified Neumann's terminology and brought attention to the developmental aspects that she considered central in understanding the representations of psychic processes that show up symbolically in sand trays.

Dora Kalff's three stages of ego development are (with the corresponding Neumann stages shown in parentheses):

1. **Animal-Vegetative Stage** (Phallic-Chthonian and Magic-Phallic): Trays that consist mainly of animals and plant life, with water and earth in the foreground. This stage represents mother-child unity
2. **Fighting/Battle Stage** (Magic-Warlike and Solar-Warlike): Trays that depict fighting and struggle. They represent the ego beginning to overcome dependence on the mother archetype and developing strong identification with the father archetype
3. **Adaption to the Collective Stage** (Solar-Rational): Trays that often include interactions among ordinary people (especially authority figures, such as parents). The scenes often take place in common settings, such as a school, zoo, or beach. These trays represent adaptation to the outer world, to the collective or group

The term "stages" refers to stages of ego development, not to steps in a sandplay process. Therefore, Kalff's stages are not necessarily sequential in sandplay. Trays that represent each of the stages may appear at several different times in a sandplay process, in various sequences. We have found that the third stage (i.e., adaptation to the collective) tends to be demonstrated more frequently toward the end of a sandplay process.

Bradway (1990) said that it was helpful for a therapist to relate the child's sand creations to the stages of ego development. She made the point that "an appreciation of what sand worlds are depicting and an empathy for the struggles and the achievements which the child encounters are conductive to providing *temenos* (Kalff's 'free and sheltered space') within which development will occur" (p.100).

The following case provides examples of trays that demonstrate Kalff's stages.

Case of Jimmy

Jimmy was referred because he was bed-wetting and was diagnosed as having primary enuresis. Up until this time, his bed-wetting hadn't seemed to bother him. However, at age seven and a half, it was beginning to affect him negatively. Friends couldn't sleep over, and when he awakened wet, he was in a foul and angry mood, and he took it out on his younger brother. According to his mother, he seemed unable to express his feelings verbally about the bed-wetting. Jimmy is quite typical of the kind of child often seen in therapy – a child that is distressed both at home and at school yet is still functioning in the world.

Jimmy was seen in almost weekly sessions for four months, followed by two more sessions at a later time period, a total of 16 sessions. During nine of his sessions, Jimmy created sandplay scenes; however, instead of having nine scenes, there are 18, because Jimmy always created two sandplay scenes – one in the dry tray and one in the wet tray. It is unusual for a child or adult to make two trays in one session, but his trays are even more unusual because of the way in which Jimmy created them: he always made them in a simultaneous manner, working on one tray for a while, then going to the other and back to the first repeatedly. Yet his two trays were not related to each other, until near the end of his therapy.

Besides the enuresis, Jimmy had problems in school – relatively small things, but things that made him something of an outsider and unable to elicit support and compassion from his teacher. For example, he went along with some other boys and pushed a girl into the boy's bathroom. Another time, he tripped a boy in line. His teacher told him to stop, but he did it again.

Some of the things his mother said about Jimmy were very revealing and relevant in understanding him, as his issues unfolded in his sand creations. His mother said that it was hard for her to really understand Jimmy and his problems because everything seemed so hidden to her. She said, with some distress in her voice, "It's hard to read Jimmy." She reported that from the beginning, he seemed to be a fussy baby who always awoke crying. This sense of discontent had continued. His mother described him as often being angry and generally unhappy with life.

Jimmy had been adopted at birth. The family had moved several times since his adoption, and they had just moved to California about five months before therapy began. His mother said that Jimmy had always seemed unusually interested in his birth parents, asking many questions about them – many more questions than his also adopted younger brother.

As Jimmy's mother told me about his background, I realized that from Jimmy's first beginnings, there had been many changes and family moves. These moves were hard on him, and he had experienced great difficulty in settling in and relaxing within his adopted family.

In Jimmy's first session, I saw a very wistful-looking, attractive Caucasian boy – not the kind of boy who catches one's heart but a more restrained and thoughtful child. During this first meeting, however, I was surprised by how articulate and self-revealing he was with me. He talked openly and freely about his bed-wetting and other feelings, including making friends and his behavior at school.

I was struck, though, with the anxiety I heard in his voice as he spoke about his birth mother and his wanting to visit her in order to ask why she had put him up for adoption. He also said that he thought she would want to see him because he believed that she wonders about what he looks like now and what he is doing. This was a very touching moment. I knew that his seeing his birth mother was not to be; Jimmy's adoption had been a very traditional one and his adopted parents had sparse information along with little motivation to be in any kind of contact with her.

During this first session, I asked him to do a Kinetic Draw-A-Family, showing his family doing something. Jimmy drew his family at the dinner table. His father and brother were in their chairs, but Jimmy could not be seen in his chair. According to him, he had dropped his knife and fork and was under the table picking them up. Also, his mother was not present at the table, even though her chair was there. Jimmy said that she had finished eating and had left the room to clean up. There was quite a lot of attention to detail: platters of food, dishes, utensils, and even napkins on the table. His small cat was nearby. It was the absence of both him and his mother from the table that set me to wondering about the solidity of the mother-child bond, in particular, and also his attachment to his family.

It was clear to me that this child was a good candidate for therapy. His family had tried many things to deal with his enuresis; however, none of these had worked, and now that Jimmy was older and more conscious, it was bothering him more and more. Also, his life-long unhappiness and discontent seemed to have infiltrated his sense of self. From the material presented by both his mother and Jimmy, I was beginning to understand the root of his long-standing unhappiness. His first sandplay and his Kinetic Draw-A-Family drawing supported these hunches.

In addition to sandplay, I also used traditional child therapy techniques with Jimmy, including play therapy, behavioral therapy, visualization, art, and bibliotherapy. Many of these techniques became appropriate as a result of looking at his sandplays and from what I learned about his life from Jimmy and his mother. There was no question that Jimmy enjoyed sandplay more than any other activity in the playroom; however, he also chose and developed other techniques that were very much in sync with the issues he illustrated in his sand creations. He loved to create sand pictures and was energetic and quick. I noticed that he enjoyed this kind of small motor activity and was quite skilled at it. I gained much understanding of Jimmy's strengths and interests by observing his work in the sand.

There is much rich imagery in his trays; however, most of this discussion will focus on those characteristics that speak to his primary issues around maternal attachment and enuresis – and demonstrations of Kalff's stages.

Figure 6.1 (Tray 1)

The first miniature Jimmy placed in the tray was a wounded man on a stretcher. Later he moved that miniature from the middle of the tray to the lifeboat in the back right. It is

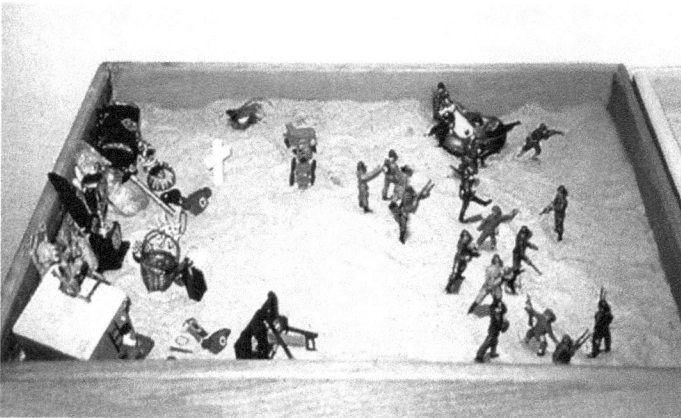

Figure 6.1 Tray 1

important to note the first item placed in a tray because sometimes that points to a direction for therapy, particularly if the item is placed in the center of a first tray.

The entire right side of the tray is occupied by soldiers, in fighting positions. In the left front corner is a cage with a tortured man inside, a time piece on the top of the cage, and a man climbing a ladder to reach the top of the cage. There also are many different miniatures on the left side, including a trophy, a tool box with tools in it, two phones separated, books, a basket of apples, a cake and candelabra by the basket, a lamp, and a large crystal with a sledgehammer against the crystal. Beside the crystal are a black arrowhead, two crowns, a treasure chest, a bird in a nest, and a cross. In the back middle is a race car.

I suspected that this child was deeply wounded, and the tortured man gave me a clue to the agony Jimmy felt. However, I also saw healing potential in the more unconscious part of the tray – the left side. The loving cup, crowns, full basket of apples, and the light that comes from the lamp and the candelabra suggest healing potential. Even though those items were not yet organized enough to be utilized, they gave me hope. The telephones suggested that communication between us was already getting established.

I was less hopeful about the empty treasure chest, the precarious crystal with the jackhammer on top, and the black arrowhead. Notice the clock with the man on the ladder trying to reach it (more about the issue of time later). The race car, a masculine symbol that suggests life energy, is present, but it is in no position to be used because there is no road.

In terms of Kalff's stages of ego development, this tray exhibits the *Fighting* stage.

Figures 6.2 and 6.3 (Tray 2)

Jimmy always worked in two sand trays at one time. This second scene, in the wet tray, was created in the same session as Tray 1. The second miniature he selected that day, a woman, was placed in the second tray. He then returned to the first tray.

Notice how quickly he was able to get organized and get going in the tray. I felt very encouraged to see what he was able to do. He created a parade led by a group of soldiers carrying flags, suggesting a sense of identity and a marching band crossing a bridge, followed by a horse-drawn golden carriage. I like to see movement in a second tray, as evidenced here;

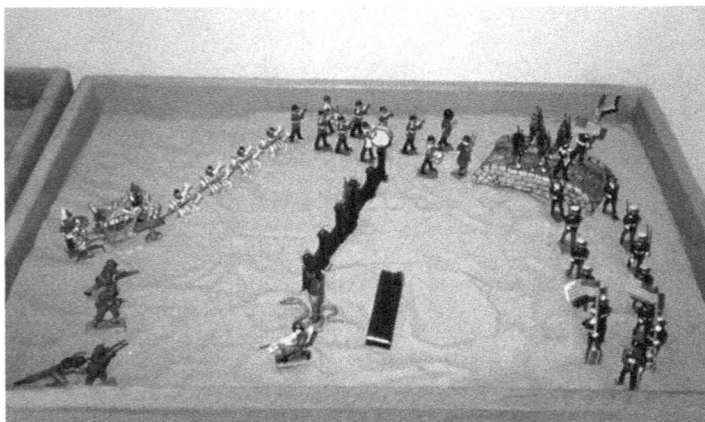

Figure 6.2 Tray 2

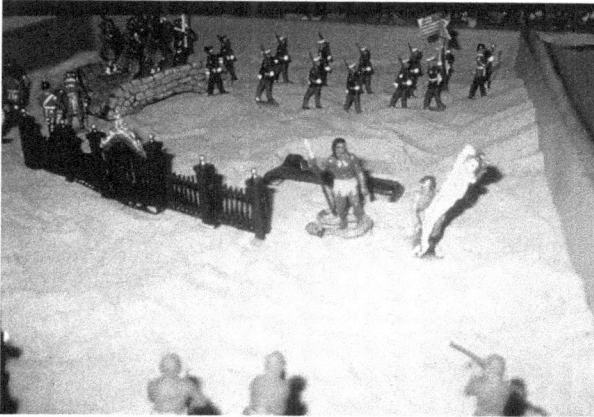

Figure 6.3 Tray 2

it is a positive sign that shows that something is getting mobilized. Again, the placement of miniatures is important. Notice that, in the front and center of the tray, he placed a nude woman next to a primitive caveman. A snake is encircling the caveman's legs. A soldier is propping up the woman (this woman was the second miniature he selected during this session). When I saw these figures, my mind immediately went to the earliest, most primitive issue of his life – that of leaving of his birth mother (mother, dad, hidden, caught in this triangle and can't develop from the primitive). This from a child who can't control his wetting.

Next, consider the stages. This is a tray that looks quite good; it is organized and activated in a positive direction. However, it has some prominent disturbing elements, e.g. the miniatures in the center (the nude woman, the snake, caveman, and soldier) reflect a prime, unresolved issue in his life – lack of bonding to his adopted family and lack of connection to the maternal. This tray best represents the *Adaptation to the Collective* stage, although in a preliminary way. His next few trays do not continue with the level of organization shown in this tray.

Figure 6.4 (Tray 3)

Two weeks later, I was surprised to see this tray and the energy that accompanied it. He used every Asian miniature I had. Once again, as he was creating this tray, he was also absorbed in making a second tray as well.

I think the reason this tray emerged at this time was that Jimmy was now able to show his chaotic internal distress and how his poorly developed ego was unable to withstand his feelings. There's much symbolism here; however, one set of items seemed particularly important: the animals from the Chinese Zodiac – a way of marking time. There was a clock in the first tray, and there were other timepieces in future trays. As a child therapist, I know that the number of therapy sessions is often controlled by the parents, especially when there is a particular identified issue, such as enuresis. In Jimmy's case, it was very obvious to me that his mother wanted his enuresis fixed quickly. Obviously, his unconscious knew that too. The chaos suggests Kalff's *Fighting* stage.

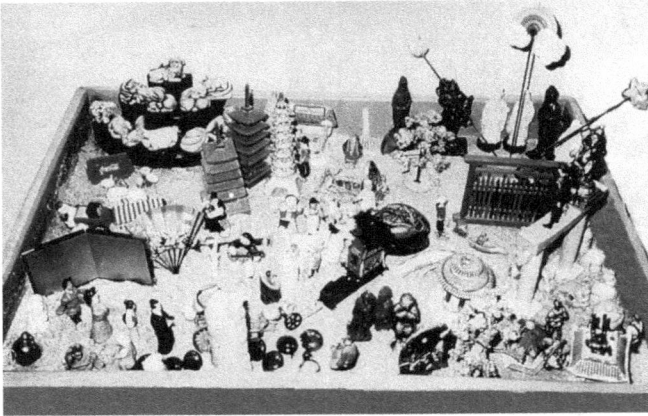

Figure 6.4 Tray 3

In this tray, he chose figures that were foreign to him; perhaps he was beginning to reach out, to explore new aspects of his potential that heretofore have been unexplored. Dora Kalff said that using images from foreign lands suggests that the client is accessing a deeper part of his/her unconscious.

Figure 6.5 (Tray 4, created the same day as Tray 3)

The many animals in this tray represent the *Animal-Vegetative* stage. However, I felt over-whelmed with all that was going on in this scene; a sense of too much pervades this tray. I began to worry about how I was going to help this child.

A few items seemed particularly important: many animals are grouped into families; how-ever, the open coffin clearly takes center stage. I wondered what had died or needed to die or

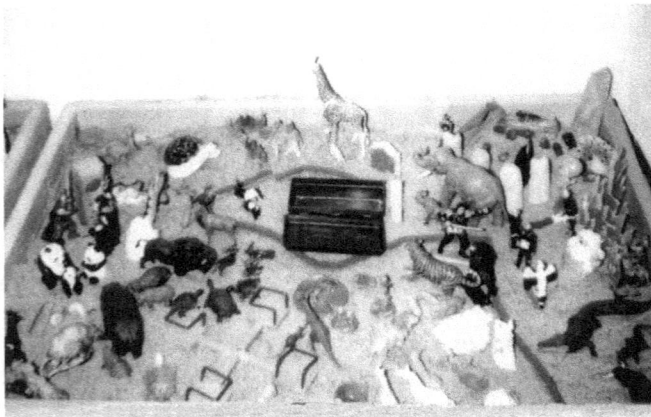

Figure 6.5 Tray 4, created the same day as Tray 3

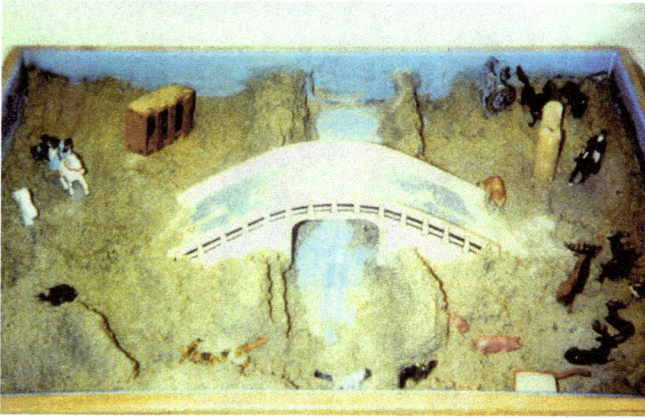

Figure 6.6 Tray 5

change. Was it his baby self that held onto wetting the bed? Was it that something inside of him was deciding which family he could attach to? Was it that he had to give up his fantasies regarding his birth mother?

Figure 6.6 (Tray 5)

I was surprised and relieved to see this tray two weeks later. Here is a new sense of organization and continuity, although still with some fragmentation. Here is a contained channel and a way to bridge over it. Jimmy put forth a great effort to make certain that the water in the channel would not spill over. After this sand picture, Jimmy spontaneously shared with me that, when he turns eight years (about six months hence), he will be ready to celebrate the end of his bed-wetting. In essence, he could visualize a time in the future when bed-wetting would be gone (dead) and forgotten as part of his self-image.

An ancient time piece is in this tray, the same one as in his first tray. Perhaps the bridge here could now serve as a connection between his birth mother and his present family. There are indications of Kalff's *Animal-Vegetative* stage. The raccoon, a nocturnal animal (the nighttime bed-wetting?), is approaching the bridge but has not as yet crossed the bridge. The mother bear is caged, and a lone turtle (a symbol of abandonment) is also contained in the tray.

Figure 6.7 (Tray 6)

In this tray, constructed the same day as Tray 5, Jimmy created an Indian village. There is an increase in life activity, and the sand picture is realistic and more unified. It appears that Jimmy is trying to develop a place for a human family, but there is still evidence of wounding and injury in the center. Yet despite this struggle, the human families have been identified. There are two family totems representing family history. Also, the families have begun to come together, as represented by the two tepees. I wondered if the question he has struggled with so long (to which family do I belong?) has finally begun to come together. Perhaps he will eventually be able to relax in his current family. Certainly, with the Indian oven

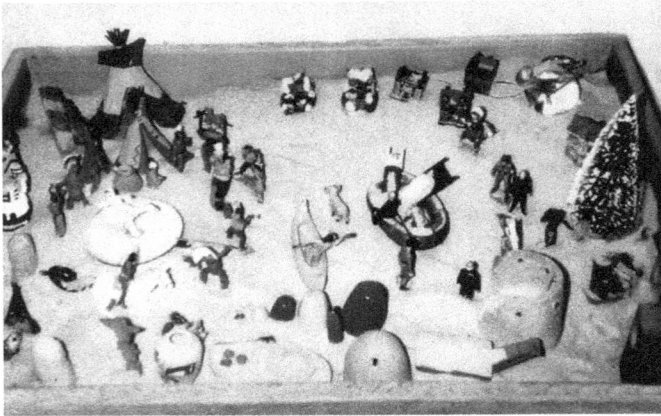

Figure 6.7 Tray 6

prominent in the tray, something is cooking and going through a process of change. This tray illustrates Kalff's *Adaptation to the Collective* stage.

With the gas pump in this tray, energy is prominent. Gas pumps have been included in previous scenes; however, he now places the pump in the lower right corner, next to where he is sitting. This suggests that his internal resources are now being activated. He now has energy to meet the struggles of his life (He will use this symbol of internal resources again as his sandplay process unfolds).

Figure 6.8 (Tray 7)

Two weeks later, here is the same bridge as used in Tray 5. Instead of the little raccoon – look at the two vehicles starting over the bridge now! There is much vitality in this tray with the

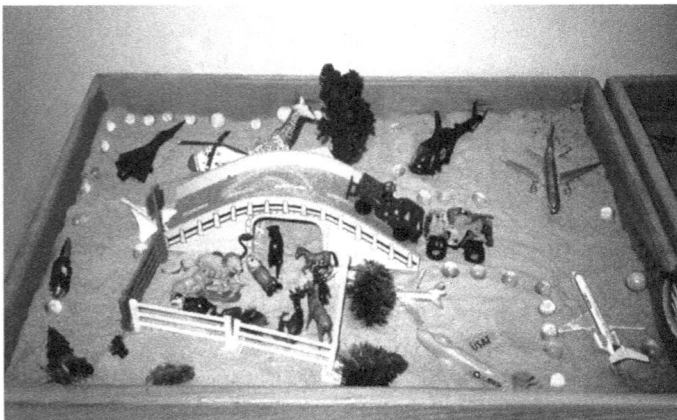

Figure 6.8 Tray 7

airplanes ready to take off. I was happy to see this alive energy, which is one of the themes suggesting movement toward wholeness. Also, there is vitality of greenery, more than in previous trays.

Bradway and McCoard (1997) wrote about the emergence of plant life in trays,

> it is an experience of self-nourishment and thus a step toward a higher level of ego autonomy. The inclusion of plant life seems to be related to an inner sense of potential for psychological growth, in contrast to the starkness of sand worlds that connote feelings of lifelessness. (p.120).

The primitive aspects are now fenced and under control. Room is made for the giraffe: the animal that is able to get above a situation in an objective way. This tray fits Kalff's *Animal-Vegetative* stage.

Figure 6.9 (Tray 8)

Note the position of the basket between the two trays (Jimmy is making this and Tray 7 at the same time). He unconsciously left one of the baskets, used to hold toys, on the edges of the two adjacent trays. Connecting the trays suggests a beginning move toward integration.

In this tray, all the army vehicles and planes look chaotic and fragmented and they suggest a struggle is going on; however, there is energy here, specifically connected to nourishment (e.g., the gas pump) and expression of natural organic growth (e.g., the trees). This suggests the *Fighting* stage. It was interesting that these two trays, created at the same session, demonstrate two very different ego stages.

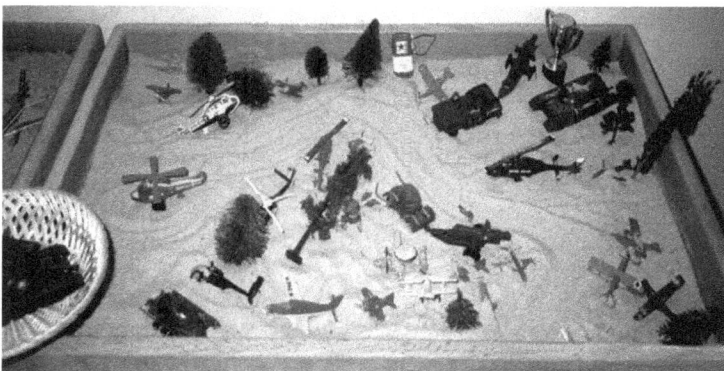

Figure 6.9 Tray 8

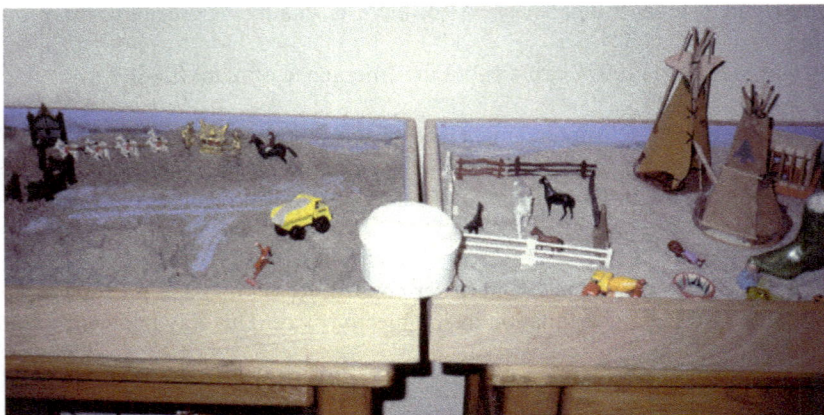

Figure 6.10 Trays 9 and 10

Figure 6.10 (Trays 9 and 10)

These trays were created two weeks later. Note the item bridging these two trays. Just as with Trays 7 and 8, Jimmy left an item unconsciously – this time it is the lid for the water container. He chose a telling symbol for his own issue of enuresis. That day he told me that he was ready to set a goal to stay dry for two weeks and we made a chart that he was going to mark himself. Perhaps now Jimmy felt more held together internally – just as the two trays are held together.

Figure 6.11 (Tray 9)

Notice the cross in the water – is this a crossroad for enuresis? Perhaps, in his gold coach, he now has a way open. The masculine car from the first tray is back, still without a road but

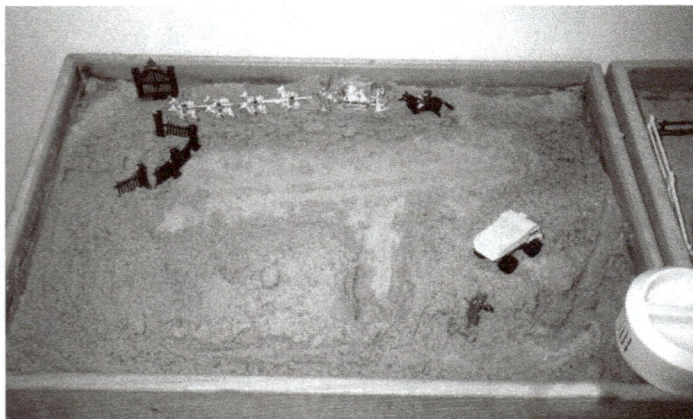

Figure 6.11 Tray 9 detail

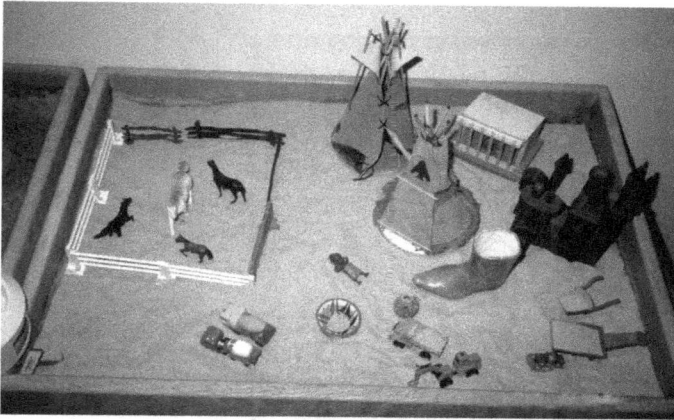

Figure 6.12 Tray 10 detail

with potential; a work machine is nearby perhaps to work on the road. A journey may be beginning.

Figure 6.12 (Tray 10)

In this tray, the masculine energies (the horses) are fenced in but with enough room to move. There are two large tepees. Perhaps this is an indication that Jimmy may eventually be able to incorporate both mothers. However, this has not happened as yet – a tepee is a home that is established but not quite settled. There is work going on with the work machines.

Note the Indian baby in the middle of the tray. Something new is emerging, but it is unattended and exposed. Jimmy's original abandonment issue may hinder the possibly of new development. I wondered if he would be able to stay in treatment long enough to receive the protection he needed or if his mother would pull him out of therapy as soon as he is dry. This is a fragile moment when new Self is beginning to constellate, as evidenced by the mandala (the bowl) and the baby. In this tray, there is an increase in life space and in realism and a somewhat more unified theme: an Indian village but with work machines. Both Trays 9 and 10 illustrate the *Adaptation to the Collective* stage.

Figure 6.13 (Tray 11, made together with Tray 12)

Just two weeks later, this is a sand scene created by an active child (not a passive one as in the previous tray). He was working very hard to get things together, and he has the means to do it (the vehicles). All the vehicles are work and rescue trucks, with boats encircling the trucks. In this picture Jimmy worked very hard to connect all the pipes; however, the job isn't done yet – just like his own plumbing. He did use all the pipes in the therapy room.

Notice the circular, contained feel of this picture. It really is a circle within a circle – certainly a clear sign of centering and coming together. This is a scene of more consolidation and integration of the self than seen before. Although it does not look as contained and defined

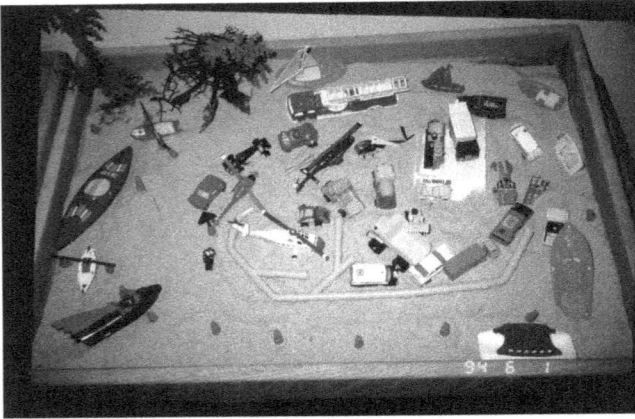

Figure 6.13 Tray 11, made together with Tray 12

as adult Self trays, the energy and joy he showed when making this tray left no doubt in my mind that this is a "Self tray." It demonstrates the *Adaptation to the Collective* stage.

Figure 6.14 (Tray 12)

Although this tray was made together with Tray 11, they are very different. Here, Jimmy went to a deeper level of the unconscious: the mother world. It is an underwater scene with shells – all symbols of the maternal depths. Recall the channel he worked on so hard to contain in Tray 5 (with the raccoon and large bridge). Now he extended the channel farther – but still

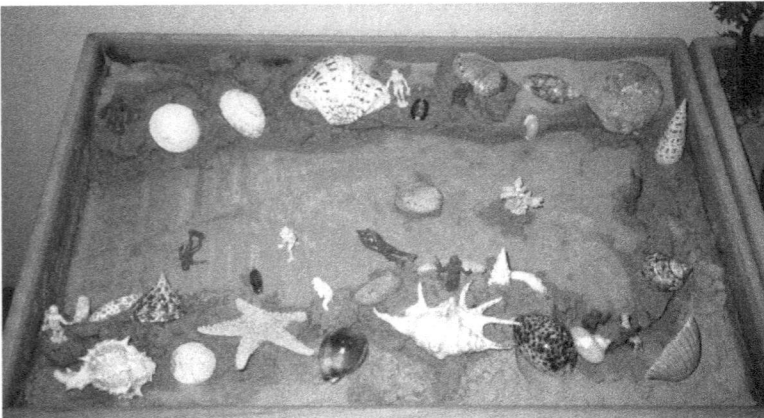

Figure 6.14 Tray 12

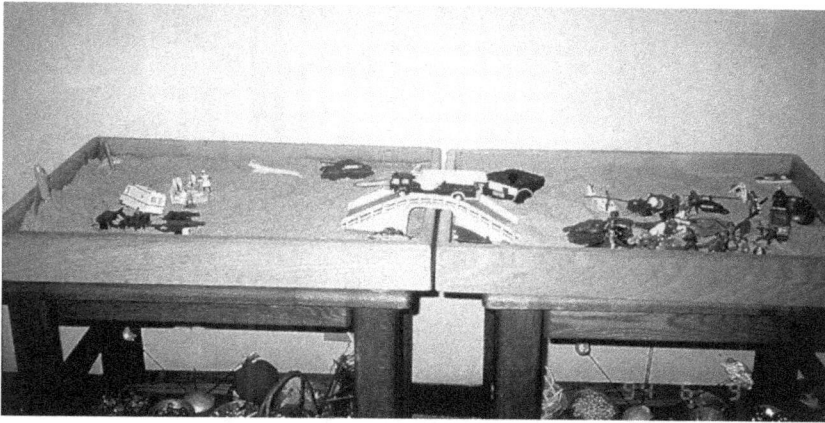

Figure 6.15 Trays 13 and 14

not quite all the way across the tray. There is a possibility that he can continue. I took special note of the starfish, a symbol of regeneration. This fits the *Animal-Vegetative* stage.

Figure 6.15 (Trays 13 and 14)

One week later, Jimmy consciously accomplished a complete bridging of two trays. For the first time, one drama encompassed both trays. Before this time, he was unable to create this much integration. Now, the struggle on the right has access and can get help from the ambulance and doctors on the left. Here, too, is a wounded man, but this time he is on a bed, surrounded by two doctors and two nurses. Jimmy told me that these airplanes (left side) were preparing to take off – and he made a path with the airplane itself as he flew the airplane into the air and back again. I wondered if this was a beginning readiness to get launched into the more grown-up world without being drawn into the regressive pull of the enuresis. At this session, Jimmy told me that he was staying dry at night, even when his mother was not getting him up to go to the bathroom.

With the appearance of the ambulance and fire truck in Tray 13, the potential of moving to Kalff's stage of *Adaptation to the Collective* is beginning. However, the fighting/struggle continues in Tray 14, which fits the *Fighting* stage.

Figure 6.16 (Tray 15, made together with Tray 16)

These trays, made one week later, demonstrate secure attachment; the cord is firmly planted in each tray. This is the kind of secure attachment that Jimmy needs to feel, regarding his place in the family and more specifically about his relationship with his mother. No longer was he the anxiously attached child that his mother described when she told me about his and her distress early in his life as she attempted to comfort him, or her feelings of not being able to understand his signals and her continued feelings of being kept distant from him. I found it very significant that Jimmy firmly anchored this cable to such a heavy base; in the outer

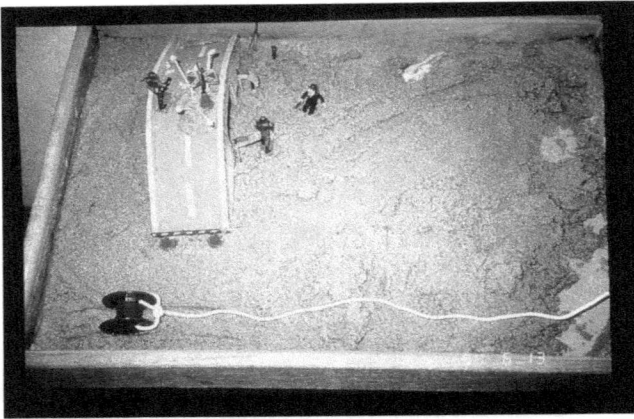

Figure 6.16 Tray 15, made together with Tray 16

world, these metal spools are so heavy that they cannot be moved easily. This cable, now securely attached, can reach all the way across.

Here, Jimmy used the same bridge he used to link Trays 13 and 14. This time it had a multitude of flags, perhaps to denote a firmer identity and sense of self. I liked the "go" sign; it could mean that he has the green light to go – take off into the world. It also could be an imperative statement reminding him what he needs to do – go to the bathroom.

Figure 6.17 (Tray 16)

Notice the cable reaches far into his other tray where a hippopotamus mother sits in the water, securely attached to her two babies. What a portrayal of how Jimmy and his younger brother

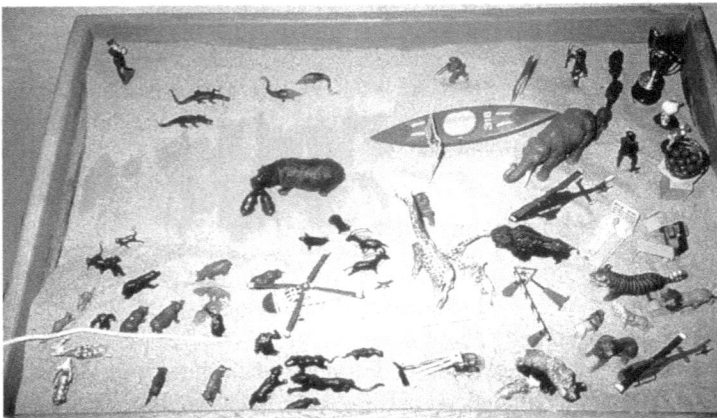

Figure 6.17 Tray 16

could now relax in the presence of the mother. Almost all the animals are now in family groupings. The wounded man is in the hospital on a bed. In Jimmy's therapy sessions, the wounded man has moved from the center of the tray to a life boat in the first tray, then to a bed-like stretcher near an ambulance with doctors in a previous tray, and now to a hospital bed, presumably recuperating. The loving cup (the trophy) appears again; this time in the right back corner. This fits the *Animal-Vegetative* stage.

After this session, Jimmy left with his family for an extended summer vacation. I had a sense that I might not see him again because he was leaving town and he was also no longer enuretic. Would his mother bring him back to therapy without this urgent problem? I was doubtful. I hoped that I would have the opportunity to help him establish himself more firmly in the world.

I saw Jimmy only two more times. The first time was in early September – three months after Tray 16. The final time was two months after that, in November. In that last session, he made a sandplay scene. During the summer he had spent much of his time with his male cousins, uncles, and Dad. He had had only one bed-wetting accident. His mother brought him back to treatment because, on his return home, his wetting began again but only infrequently. During the September session he did not use the sand tray.

He created his last two trays in our concluding session, the session in November. He knew that it would be his last session with me. He told me that he had only wet the bed twice since he saw me in September and that he didn't need to see me because he was now dry. However, he wanted to say goodbye. This session was right before his eighth birthday. Recall that he said he would celebrate his staying dry on that birthday. We both knew that it was not possible to convince his parents of continuing therapy.

Jimmy also told me that school was going well and he liked his teacher this year much better than last year's teacher, who he knew didn't like him. He was actively involved with six other boys, including his younger brother, in building a tree house in the neighborhood. He shared a poem he had written that had to do with the rain that would come in spring to nurture the flowers. I heard this communication as telling me about the renewal of his own energy and life force. Water moved from having earlier been his nemesis in the bed-wetting, to now having found its proper place, that of nurturing and renewal.

Figures 6.18-6.20 (Trays 17 and 18)

Here are his final trays. Although they could be viewed separately, it is important to realize that Jimmy created one integrated picture, using both trays. Now, there is a realistic, organized, and unified theme that covers the whole of the two trays. No longer is a bridge needed to integrate the trays. He began by asking permission to move some of the wet sand into the dry tray – perhaps a move of integration. Taken together, both trays show "a day at the zoo." Clearly, this represents *Adaptation to the Collective*.

These last two trays are his statement about his making it in the ordinary world. Notice, for the first time, he used only present-day, ordinary people. In both trays there is an observing ego: the families watching the animals. He can now stand back and observe because the animals are fenced in. As the wild animals are fenced in, he is better able to fence his own primitive needs and impulses. His enuresis was under control, and he could take his place in the everyday world at school and at home. He was a more agreeable, relaxed child to live with.

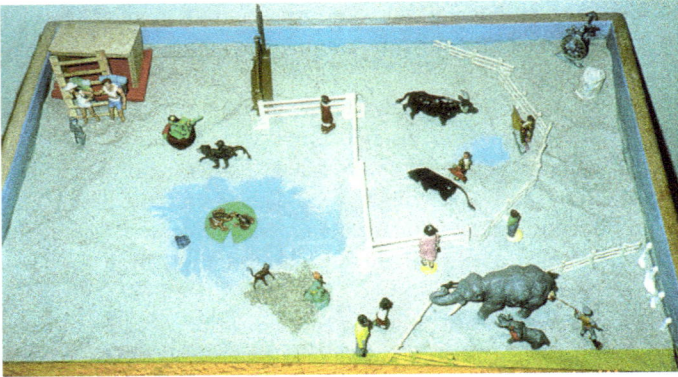

Figure 6.18 Tray 17

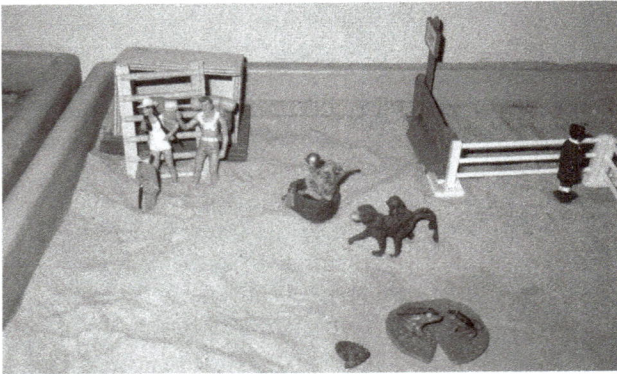

Figure 6.19 Tray 17 detail

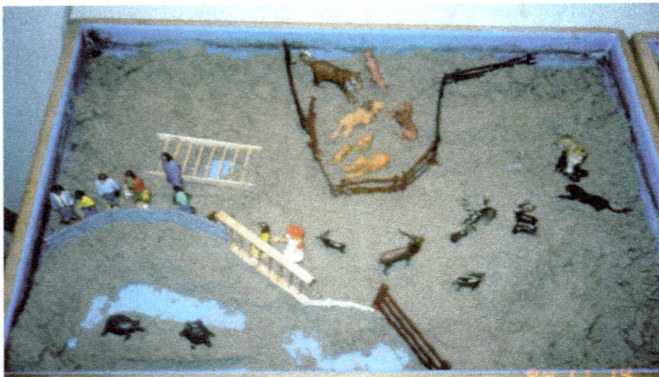

Figure 6.20 Tray 18

Three Stages of Ego Development
Jimmy's Sandplay Journey

STAGE	1	2	3	4	5	6	7	8	9	10	11	12	13/14	15/16	17/18
Animal-Vegetative	X		X	X		X					X			X	
Fighting Stage (Struggle)		X						X					X	X	
Adaptation To Collective	X				X				X	X	X				X

Figure 6.21 Table summarizing Jimmy's trays

The two frogs on the round lily pad create a lovely image. Frogs go through more life cycle stages than any other animal. However, there still may be work to be done. The turtle is a symbol of abandonment because after the mother turtle lays her eggs, she leaves the eggs alone and unprotected to hatch and make the perilous trip into the water. Here is Jimmy's statement that he has almost been able to make this trip into the water – but not quite. Yet he is accompanied on the trip by another turtle. Perhaps this speaks to the transference.

Figure 6.21

This table summarizes Jimmy's sandplay journey and the main demonstrations of the Kalff stages. Note several characteristics: (a) all three of the stages were seen in his trays; (b) the stages appeared several times and were not necessarily sequential; and (c) Kalff's *Adaptation to the Collective* stage was apparent in trays at several points in his process, and was very prominent in his final session.

Jimmy was no longer enuretic; we had reached the goal his parents had for him. Yet I also thought he still had issues regarding his abandonment by his birth mother. I felt pleased about Jimmy's new integration, his relaxation in the family, and the bonding with the other family members, as seen in the last tray. What a contrast his last tray was with the chaotic and wounded trays he created in the beginning. He had come a long way.

References

Bradway, K. (1990). Development stages in children's sand worlds. In K. Bradway, K. Signell, G. Spare, C. Stewart, L. Stewart, & C. Thompson (Eds.), *Sandplay studies: Origins, theory and practice* (2nd ed., pp. 93–100). Sigo Press.

Bradway, K., & McCoard, B. (1997). *Sandplay: Silent workshop of the psyche*. Routledge.

Kalff, D. (1980). *Sandplay: A psychotherapeutic approach to the psyche* (W. Ackerman, Trans.). Sigo Press. (Originally published, 1966, in German as Sandspiel by Rascher. First published, 1971, in English as Sandplay: Mirror of a child's psyche (H. Kirsch, Trans.) by Browser Press).

Neumann, E. (1990). *The child* (R. Manheim, Trans.). Shambhala.

Chapter 7

Tracking themes in sandplay therapy

A most useful way to understand sandplay scenes, as well as the sandplay process, is to track the changes in clients' sandplay pictures. For many years, we studied our clients' sandplay scenes to identify the types of changes we saw in the scenes over time. Gradually, we began to see common patterns emerging, and we followed our visual and cognitive reactions when we began to both identify and organize those patterns.

We observed that specific themes repeated themselves. After further study, we found that it was possible to cluster these themes into two groups: themes of wounding and themes of healing. We eventually realized that the themes were archetypal patterns that appear during a sandplay process and that these patterns are inborn, unconscious, archetypal structures residing within all human beings. From this research, we realized that tracking the themes is helpful in following the movement in sandplay therapy, as well as observing a client's stage of development and therapeutic progress.

Specific themes can be identified in almost all sandplay scenes, and some themes are likely to be present throughout a client's entire series. For example, it is somewhat common for the theme denoting "energy" to be present in multiple trays with miniatures portraying work machines and/or organic growth. Other themes may be expressed dramatically and then never reappear.

Defining sandplay themes

A sandplay theme is a visual image or set of images in a sandplay picture. Identifying themes in clients' trays over time can help clinicians and researchers to: (a) understand clients' current issues and psychic state; (b) monitor psychological change and growth; (c) determine effectiveness of therapy; and (d) communicate, when appropriate, clients' current issues, as well as changes in development and growth over time.

Based on observations and findings from clinical study conducted by the authors, we found that, as therapy progresses, fewer wounding themes will be present in sandplay pictures and more healing themes will emerge. Further, we found that:

- Themes can be found in almost all sandplay pictures
- Each sandplay picture may contain a number of themes
- Themes cluster naturally into two groups – themes of wounding and themes of healing

Themes of wounding appear most often in trays of clients who:

- Had early abuse, trauma, illness, loss or death of family member
- Are in the early stages of therapy

Themes of healing appear most often in trays of clients who:

- Had healthy, less traumatic early environments
- Are in the latter stages of therapy

As therapy progresses, both wounding and healing themes change quantitatively and qualitatively. In the early phases of therapy, sandplay pictures usually contain more themes of wounding than of healing. As therapy progresses, more themes of healing and wholeness emerge and eventually outnumber themes of wounding. In the latter stages of therapy, themes of wounding become:

- Less prominent, smaller, or simplified
- More disconnected or fragmented and less integrated into the scene
- Changed in positive ways

As therapy progresses, themes of healing become:

- More prominent, enlarged, or enriched
- More realistic or life-like
- Less disconnected or fragmented and more integrated into the entire scene

Each of the 20 themes (ten wounding themes and ten healing themes) is defined and described below. These themes were identified through our current research (additional themes may be added in the future).

Examples of each theme (based on actual sandplay scenes created by children and adults) are included to illustrate various types and levels of clarity. In addition, key psychological implications for each theme are provided in order to assist clinicians in identifying possible meanings for a client's use of specific themes.

The material in this section is based on our clinical experience in observing the themes used by our own clients. This section is not meant to be inclusive of all possible interpretations. We have, however, attempted to include a wide range of possible meanings.

Specific coding examples are presented below for each of the themes, using the following point system:

0 points = Theme is not evident
1 point = Theme is present
2 points = Theme is prominent

Coding themes in sandplay scenes requires judgment, experience, and psychological acumen. Normally, prominence and/or clear evidence of a theme in a sandplay scene are the primary considerations in determining the point coding. However, at times, the developmental level of a client has to be taken into account. For example, a young child's tray that looks chaotic actually may be a result of age-appropriate coordination difficulties, rather than internal disorganization.

Examples of possible long-term and short-term behavioral goals are included to assist the clinician in developing clinical goals based on themes in client's sandplay pictures. As the themes move from wounding to healing, the goal descriptions change to communicate increased development and growth.

Wounding themes

Wounding themes appear most often in the early stages of therapy and suggest that trauma and/ or some type of wounding has occurred. However, sandplay scenes of children under eight years, who have not experienced trauma, may also contain these themes, because of their lack of physical and mental ability to create anything other than a picture with wounding themes.

1. Chaotic tray: A chaotic, undifferentiated or amorphous tray. The arrangement seems haphazard, fragmented, or formless
   Examples:

- Objects are flung into the tray
- Boundaries or outer reality disregarded
- Items are carefully placed, but the overall appearance is jumbled or disconnected

Possible psychological implications:

- Reflection of chaos in client's external world
- A display of internal disorganization
- Overwhelming and/or conflicted feelings
- An inability to contain the opposites
- Letting go of too restrictive controls
- Disintegration preceding new integration
- For young children, may be age appropriate
- For adults, may be an indicator of early wounding, anger, terror, or a lifelong issue

Coding:

0 = Chaotic theme not evident
1 = Items are placed carefully and, for the most part, are upright, but the overall appearance appears jumbled or disconnected
2 = Little care is taken in placement of objects and tray is disorganized and/or overfilled with items; the tray's boundaries are disregarded (Also code 2 if a large pile of toys without a theme is present)

Short-term behavioral goals; client is able to:

- Identify the source of distress
- Decrease frequency of impulsive acts
- Learn how to deal with overwhelming feelings
- Enlist familial help to lessen stressful situations

Long-term behavioral goals; client is able to:

- Differentiate issues and consider possible solutions
- Come to terms with early trauma
- Effectively channel impulses

2. **Empty or barren tray**: An empty tray, reticence to use figures, a lifeless feeling with a lack of energy and curiosity
Examples:

- Client may move the sand, but does not follow through by placing miniatures in the tray
- Empty or nearly empty tray with a single object placed in a corner
- Sometimes miniatures are spread over the entire tray yet few miniatures are used

Possible psychological implications:

- Lack of internal or external freedom of expression
- Discomfort in accessing and/or displaying aspects of the unconscious
- Unconscious attempt to hide aspects of him/herself
- Ego strength may not be strong or differentiated enough to make a personal statement
- Possible depression
- Discomfort or lack of trust in the transference
- Making space for new development

Coding:

0 = Empty theme not evidenced
1 = Lifeless feeling with lack of energy
2 = Empty or nearly empty tray (tray is at least three-quarters empty)

Short-term behavioral goals:

- Increase sense of self-acceptance
- Increase freedom to express oneself
- Feel freer to expose self

Long-term behavioral goals:

- Increase ability to express self
- Increase awareness of self
- Increase ego strength
- Develop a consistent, positive self-image

3. **Split or barricaded**: Parts of the tray are separated or detached; figures or groupings of figures are isolated from one another

Examples:

- River, road, fence, sand, or objects divide the tray
- Miniatures are placed end to end, dividing the tray

Possible psychological implications:

- Difficulty in containing opposites
- Defense against overwhelming feelings
- Unconscious dissociation
- A new separation from old patterns
- A sorting out, differentiating oneself from others

Coding:

0 = Split theme not evidenced
1 = Slight split
2 = A clearly defined split or division in tray; divide goes across tray (Also code if a river, road, fence, or row of miniatures divide the tray)

Short-term behavioral goals:

- Identify key issues in alienated state

Long-term behavioral goals:

- Integrate aspects of personality

4. **Confined**: Miniatures that are normally free are entrapped or caged
Examples:

- An agonized human figure is placed in a cage
- A sand wall is built around an old woman

Possible psychological implications

- An unconscious effort to hide aspects of themselves
- A lack of internal and/or external freedom of expression
- An attempt to restrict frightening or menacing elements
- Unsafe feelings in current environment
- Creating boundaries for protection/self-control

Coding:

0 = Confined theme not evidenced
1 = Element of confinement
2 = Confinement dominates the tray (people are enclosed by fences, walls, or boxes)

Short-term behavioral goals:

- Identify issues that are hindering growth

Long-term behavioral goals:

- Client is less constrained
- Key life conflicts and emotional stress that cause constrictive patterns are resolved

5. **Neglected**: A figure appears isolated from possible support or protection; help is unavailable to a figure in need
Examples:

- Baby is left in a high chair while mother is sleeping in another room
- Child or baby appears abandoned
- Lone soldier is facing enemy while companions have their backs to him/her

Possible psychological implications:

- Abandonment during early development
- Feelings of abandonment in current relationships
- Lack of awareness and care of one's own needs
- An attack on the Self

Coding:

0 = Neglected theme not evidenced
1 = Feeling of neglect
2 = Clear evidence of neglect

Short-term behavioral goals:

- Identify people in client's current life who would be willing to support and protect client

Long-term behavioral goals:

- Learn how to support and protect self

6. **Hidden**: Figures are buried or hidden from view
Examples:

- Gun is hidden behind a house
- A watch is buried in the sand under a tree
- Client buries an object in the sand to hide it from the therapist
- Client hides an object from other miniatures in the tray

Possible psychological implications:

- Resistance or inability to look at or deal with life issues
- Lack of trust in self and others
- Insufficient ego strength to deal with current life issues
- Reluctance to deal with disturbing feelings
- Early life pattern of hiding from life challenges
- Age-appropriate playful behavior

Coding:

0 = Hidden theme not evidenced
1 = Items hidden behind other objects
2 = Items hidden in the sand

Short-term behavioral goals:

- Build ego strength
- Openly deal with life challenges
- Become more trusting of others
- Become more able to deal with life challenges

Long-term behavioral goals:

- Be able to understand and deal with life issues
- Realistically deal with reality
- Become more open and trusting of others

7. **Prone**: Figures that are normally upright are placed, consciously or unconsciously, in a reclining or fallen position
Examples:

- A standing pregnant woman is placed face down in the sand
- Two galloping deer are placed on their sides

Psychological implications:

- Indication of early wounding
- Mindful of photographic effect; wants figure viewed from side, rather than from the top
- Possible indicator of an undiagnosed physical issue
- Insufficient ego strength

Coding:

0 = Prone theme not evidenced
1 = Items left prone in the process of play. e.g., cat falls out of tree and is left in sand
2 = Items intentionally placed in prone position, e.g., baby placed laying in bathtub

(Code 2 if animals or people are face down in sand)

Short-term behavioral goals:

- Identify and be able to discuss early psychological issues
- Be alert to possibility of physical health issues

Long-term behavioral goals:

- Build ego strength
- Resolution of early psychological issues
- Feeling of physical and psychological well-being

8. **Injured**: Figures are injured or in the process of being harmed
Examples:

- Bandaged man lying on a stretcher
- A cowboy placed in the mouth of a dinosaur

Possible psychological implications:

- Suggests current or past psychic injury, perhaps at an early age
- Defense against overwhelming feelings
- Possible physical or psychological issue that needs immediate attention
- An old injury needing attention is exposed

Coding:

0 = Injured theme not evidenced
1 = Incidental injury
2 = Clear evidence of an injury; intended injury (Code 2 if a wounded figure is used)

Short-term behavioral goals:

- Identify disturbing issues

Long-term behavioral goals:

- Repair old wounds

9. **Threatened**: Menacing or frightening events are happening in the tray and the endangered figure(s) are unable to deal with the experience. Shadow material is predominant and overwhelming
Examples:

- Aggressive animals are surrounding a small child
- One army is significantly more powerful than another army

Psychological implications:

- Insufficient ego strength to meet life issues
- Fear of moving through life stages
- Feelings of being overwhelmed and insufficient

Coding:

0 = Threatened theme not evidenced
1 = Passive threat
2 = Active threat (Code 2 if vulnerable miniature is surrounded or threatened by aggressive miniatures)

Short-term behavioral goals:

- Become less fearful of others
- Be able to meet transitions in life with more ease
- Become less defensive with others

Long-term behavioral goals:

- Become more able to trust others
- Develop ego strength
- Feel less overwhelmed in meeting life issues

10. **Hindered**: Threatening events appear prominent and hinder or impede the possibility of new growth
Examples:

- A beautiful or centered sandplay that contains one or more elements that could over-shadow and curtail moving forward
- A boat trying to move into new waters while threatened by distant soldiers with guns pointed at the boat
- A person, walking along a path in a lovely garden, seems to be unaware that a snake is buried nearby

Psychological implications:

- Unconscious awareness of shadow elements
- Defense against looking at the larger picture
- New growth is being threatened by cultural and family archetypal patterns
- Natural resistance to new developments

Coding:

0 = Hindered theme not evidenced
1 = Fencing without a gate or other impediments; slightly hindered
2 = Dramatic or active impediments (Code when path or activity is impeded)

Short-term behavioral goals:

- Increase ability to meet development life stages

Long-term behavioral goals:

- Meet life challenges with ease
- Increase ability to deal realistically with life issues

Healing themes

These themes appear more often in latter phases of therapy, suggesting that the process is moving in the direction of healing, wholeness, and transformation.

1. **Bridging**: A physical connection is made between two or more elements in the tray. The capacity to connect elements, bridge the opposites, or connect the conscious and unconscious elements in the tray
Examples:

- A ladder joins earth and tall trees
- A bridge links an angel and a devil
- A rainbow is placed between a body of water and the sand

Possible psychological implications:

- Resolution of the opposites
- Indicates new internal potential beyond the conscious mind
- Marrying of opposites, which has (as its fruition) the birth of a new element
- New connection is made between two previously opposing issues

Coding:

0 = Bridging theme not evidenced
1 = Bridging aspects present but no clear opposites
2 = Bridging joining opposites (Code 2 when a bridge is used or created)

Short-term behavioral goals:

- Able to connect to new ideas and others
- Able to think in a more organized manner

Long-term behavioral goals:

- Open to new information and ideas
- Ability to actualize new ideas in the world
- Works cooperatively with others
- Increase sense of well-being

2. **Journeying**: Movement along a path or around a center, toward wholeness
Examples:

- Walking unhindered along a path, following a trail, circular movements around a center
- Native American paddles a canoe down a stream

Possible psychological implications:

- Awareness that something new and larger beckons
- The possibility of a departure from known and old behavior
- An awareness of necessity of giving up old behavior
- Acceptance of the reality of the greater internal self

Coding:

0 = Journeying theme not evidenced
1 = Element of Journeying
2 = Journeying predominates tray (Code 2 when vehicle moves down path)

Short-term behavioral goals:

- Experimenting with new behaviors

Long-term behavioral goals:

- Replacing some old behaviors with new, improved ones

3. **Energized**: An alive, focused, and intense energy appears, suggesting readiness to respond and move out into the world
Examples:

- Organic growth is present
- Construction machines work on a task
- Airplanes take off

Possible psychological implications:

- Healing energy is becoming activated
- A stronger, developing ego
- An increased ability to deal with the outer world
- Connection to one's own natural abilities
- A state of mania

Coding:

0 = Energy theme not evidenced
1 = Energy is an aspect of tray
2 = Energy dominates tray (Code 2 when green trees, plants, or airplanes are used)

Short-term behavioral goals

- Has increased ability to deal with daily life issues

Long-term behavioral goals:

- Has sufficient energy to meet life challenges

4. **Going Deeper**: An image of encountering the depths, discovering a deeper dimension and accessing healing powers of the unconscious
Examples:

- A clearing is made
- A treasure is unearthed
- A well is dug
- A lake is created or explored
- A natural disaster occurs, such as a tornado or flood, and creates a new landscape

Possible psychological implications:

- Hidden, internal abilities are accessed
- Old, destructive patterns are less prominent allowing new positive energy to emerge
- An increased awareness of the internal Self and one's fuller potential
- An ability to experience the numinous and be on a path toward individuation
- This process may lead toward the creation of a "Self" tray

Coding:

0 = Going Deeper theme not evidenced
1 = Going Deeper is an aspect of the tray
2 = Going Deeper predominates the tray (Code when submarine, fisherman, or diver are used, if a buried treasure is found)

Short-term behavioral goals:

- Becoming more introspective

Long-term behavioral goals:

- New internal abilities are developed

5. **Birthing**: Emergence of new development and potential for healing
Examples:

- A baby is born
- A flower opens
- A bird incubates eggs

Possible psychological implications:

- A new awareness is now possible
- New behaviors are possible
- Increased consciousness
- Increased ability to reflect and think about oneself
- Compensation for a sense of deadness

Coding:

0 = Birthing theme not evident
1 = Birth initiated but not completed, e.g., seeds buried
2 = Birthing enacted (Code 2 if actual birth scene or baby sits on stone or on mother)

Short-term behavioral goals:

- Becoming more introspective

Long-term behavioral goals:

- New internal abilities are developed

6. **Nurturing**: Nourishment and/or help appears to support growth and development
Examples:

- A mother feeds a baby
- Supportive family groups gather
- A nurse helps a patient
- Food is present

Possible psychological implications:

- Internal support is available for development
- External support (positive transference) is available for development
- Ability to connect to internal/external resources
- Connections to positive energies possible
- Feeling that needs can be satisfied
- Increased ability to trust
- A substitute for internal and external nourishment

Coding:

0 = Nurturing theme not evidenced
1 = Use of food or other nurturing items
2 = Nurturing is acted out, e.g., baby is fed (Code 2 if food is present)

Short-term behavioral goals:

- Increase trust
- Accept external support

Long-term behavioral goals:

- Internal and external resources cause needs to be satisfied

7. **Changed**: Sand and/or miniatures are changed, moved, stacked, and/or contoured as an essential part of the picture
Examples:

- Sand is contoured to build a land bridge
- Sand is moved or stacked as an essential part of the sand picture
- House is built from twigs picked up on walk to school

Possible psychological implications:

- Imaginative use of inner resources
- Positive prognosis
- Indicates an ability to make changes
- Creative capacity
- A frenetic manipulation of sand in search of control

Coding:

0 = Changed theme not evidenced
1 = Items or sand changed in ways congruent with the object, e.g., sand pushed aside to create
    lake, transformer figure used in picture
2 = Items or sand are creatively changed or used (Code if sand is moved significantly or if an
    object is used in a way different from that intended)

Short-term behavioral goals:

- Begin making selected changes

Long-term behavioral goals:

- Make significant changes

8. **Spiritual elements**: Religious and spiritual symbols are present
Examples:

- Supernatural beings, worshiping figures, or numinous representations of nature are
  present

- Buddha overlooking a newly married couple
- Creation of a sacred space

Possible psychological implications:

- Ability to access the depths of one's internal life
- Ability to experience a larger dimension of life
- Ability to see beyond one's own ego state
- Ability to experience the numinous
- A flight away from everyday life

Coding:

0 = Spiritual theme not evidenced
1 = Religious and spiritual symbols present in tray
2 = Religious and spiritual symbols predominate tray (Code if religious figures are used)

Short-term behavioral goals:

- Experience some broader aspects of life

Long-term behavioral goals:

- Find broader, greater meaning in life

9. **Centered**: A tray that contains a circular shape or a central gathering in which elements are aesthetically balanced or a union of opposites
Examples:

- Wedding couple is placed in the center of the tray
- Mandala is centered in the tray
- Round lake or round mound is near the middle of the tray

Possible psychological implications:

- A state of union is possible or has been achieved
- Psychic split has been healed
- (Jung interpreted the mandala as an expression of the psyche and, in particular, the Self)
- Potential for wholeness
- Can be used defensively for those who are fragmented

Coding:

0 = Centered theme not evidenced
1 = Elements are esthetically balanced in the center of the tray, or a union of opposites occurs
    with extraneous objects present
2 = Mandala or centering predominates tray (Code if the tray is only one congruent scene)

Short-term behavioral goals:

- Thinks more clearly
- Behaves in appropriate ways in the world

Long-term behavioral goals:

- Client is more at ease with self and others

10. **Integrated**: Contains a congruent, organized scene encompassing the entire tray. This unity of expression suggests wholeness and integration
Examples:

- A zoo encompasses the entire tray
- A baseball game covers the entire tray
- An abstract construction unifies the entire tray

Possible psychological implications:

- Ability to withstand the tension of the opposites
- Integration of the opposites
- A necessary process for individuation
- Holding various aspects of the personality providing a sense of wholeness
- Defense against an inner sense of chaos

Coding:

0 = Integrated theme not evidenced
1 = One scene, a town or village, partially unified
2 = Whole scene is completely integrated (Code if there is a single congruent scene)

Short-term behavioral goals:

- Reports feeling more at ease in the world and with others
- More accepting of self and others
- Is able to use the environment in appropriate and realistic ways

Long-term behavioral goals:

- Behaves in a predictable and congruent manner
- Words and actions go together
- Congruent behavior with others
- Has joyful attitude toward life

Examples of sandplay themes in Tammy's process

Tammy was 37 years old when she began therapy. She had been divorced three years and was still attempting to find her way in the world as a single woman. She immediately communicated her feelings of dissatisfaction with her current life, her two teenage children, both her women and men friends, and ultimately dissatisfaction with herself.

She was born and brought up on the Eastern seaboard where many wealthy generations of family had lived before, including servants who worked for and supported the family. The family tradition included a special nanny for each child who looked after each of the children's daily needs as they grew up.

Tammy was the only girl in the family with four older brothers. She was the long-awaited girl. It was hard for her mother to give this child away to a nanny so soon after her birth. In this family's tradition, she did so but reluctantly. Mother's envy and rivalry with the nanny for Tammy's affection was always present and continued to remain a lifelong issue. On one side there was a loving mother and on the other side a nanny who was deeply attached and committed, with a strong need to win Tammy's love away from her mother. Because of this confusing situation, Tammy grew up unable to fully relax in the arms of either of these women, and she felt caught in their ongoing rivalry. Another important but much more hidden factor was an unavailable narcissistic father, sometimes in the background but also in the foreground of this family drama.

Tammy's internal feeling reality in the family was that Dad was present for the brothers but not for her. He was away on business often or, when at home, mostly spent time with her brothers and rarely with Tammy. He ran his powerful family business with a tyrannical, iron hand. Tammy heard the servants refer him to him as "a devil" or "the demon king of the house." It became increasingly clear that Tammy had been deprived of an experience of embodied fathering, never having had a chance to grow her own natural masculinity.

The sand trays that Tammy made depict both the negative, destructive relationship she had in her internal world and her inner potential that eventually emerged for healing. You will see Tammy's developing ego that eventually allowed her to meet her life challenges. These 15 trays are only some of those she created over the years but are numbered as 15 for convenience.

Figure 7.1 (Tray 1)

Tammy seemed very tense when she created her first tray. She first drew two circles in the sand and said, "I feel like I have two separate life stories in my heart, and I have carried these two stories forever and they could never touch." She also talked about how alone she had always been and that no one was ever really there for her. According to Dora Kalff, the therapist's initial feeling response to a tray (especially the first tray) needs to be honored and included in understanding what is pictured in the tray. The therapist felt very sad when viewing this tray. The *Empty* and *Split* themes are very prominent in this tray, therefore each theme is scored two points.

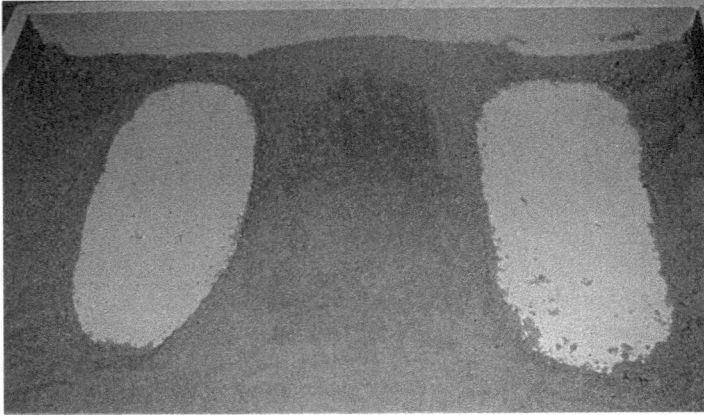

Figure 7.1 Tray 1

Figure 7.2 (Tray 2)

A few months later – splitting in the trays has continued, with some slight changes – this tray resembles a worried baby looking directly out into the world. Notice the change in her use of the two circles and her increasing ability to change the sand. It is still *Split*, and somewhat *Empty*, but she is now *Changing* and using the sand creatively – this takes energy. This is her first healing theme.

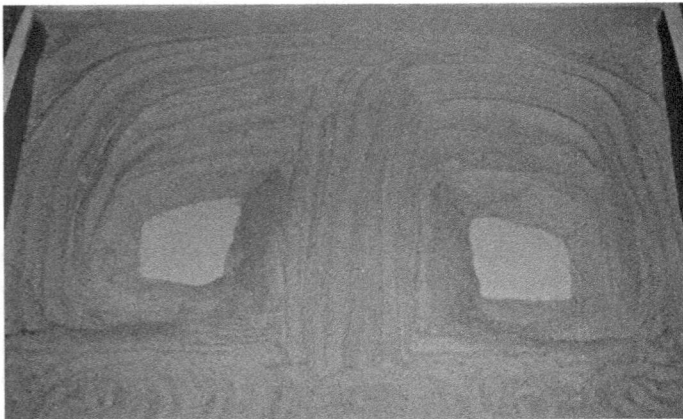

Figure 7.2 Tray 2

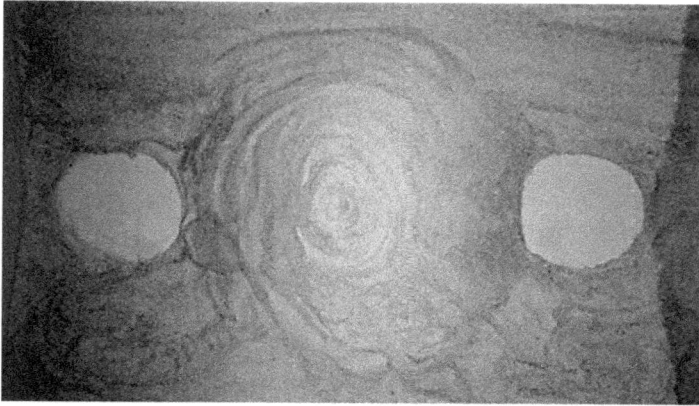

Figure 7.3 Tray 3

Figure 7.3 (Tray 3)

Split but *Centered* and *Energized*: almost a year later, a large mound emerges to bridge two circles, which are decreasing in size. The therapist wondered what unconscious contents were trying to "push up" toward the light of consciousness, or what might be cooking inside her that might be able to bridge this long-standing split.

Figures 7.4 and 7.5 (Tray 4)

After 18 months of Tammy creating many split trays, the therapist began to wonder if more change was possible. This tray was created nine months after the previous tray. While the theme of splitting continues, now – for the first time – a connection is made. The tray begins to look more human, perhaps; it is a face. At the point where the sides of the V touch, she

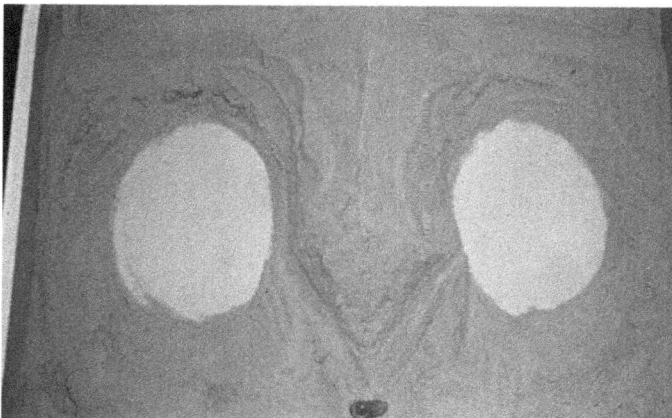

Figure 7.4 Tray 4

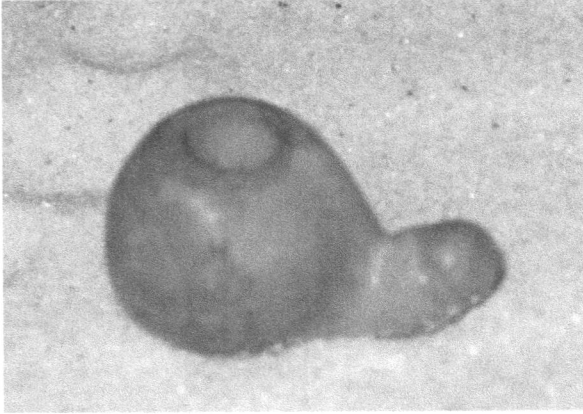

Figure 7.5 Tray 4 detail

places the first miniature she has ever used. It is a small phallus, placed right between the two circles and at the bottom of the V.

The therapist thought at this moment, "This is just what she needs to bridge – the great divide about her father." Tammy suffered from father hunger, never feeling she had enough of her dad. She yearned for him to rescue her from the rivalry of the two moms (her mother and nanny). Tammy's psyche came up with exactly what she so desperately needed – masculine energy. However, a prominent *Split* continues in this tray, but she has changed the sand in a creative way. So, this tray contains a *Changed* healing theme as well as a split theme.

Figure 7.6 (Tray 5)

Now, for the first time, Tammy moves the sand with much more freedom, more like a young child free to experiment and make a mess with the sand. She worked a long time to create this

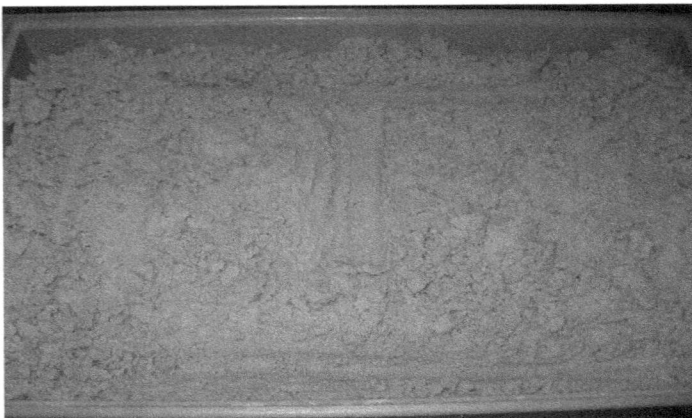

Figure 7.6 Tray 5

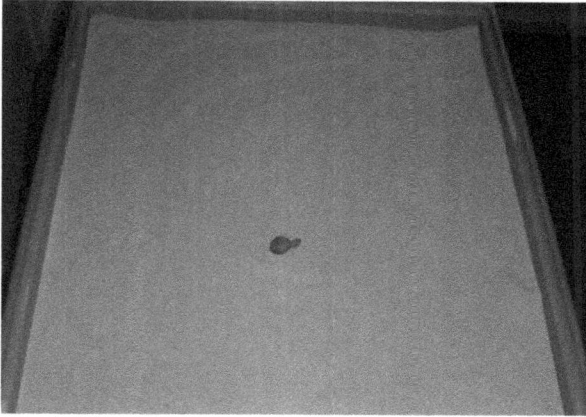

Figure 7.7 Tray 6

tray – her first one without any separate circles. While making the tray she kept asking, "Am I boring you; am I taking too long?" However, with reassurance that it was OK, she continued working. Notice the emergence of an outline of a cross.

This tray is *Chaotic* – a haphazard or formless arrangement (2 points); it is also *Split*, but the split is not prominent – therefore one point.

Figure 7.7 (Tray 6)

Now, different kinds of trays begin to emerge. This time, Tammy used the entire tray and quickly smoothed the sand. Then once again, she placed the same small phallus that she had used in Tray 4, in the center of the tray. The prominent wounding theme is an *Empty* tray – a reticence to use figures.

Figures 7.8 and 7.9 (Tray 7)

There are two healing themes in this tray, *Centered* and *Energized* (the green trees) with no wounding themes present.

Now we see what has emerged from the initial split, the chaos, and the emptiness of the earlier trays. From this narrow and self-centered world, a hand reaches toward the heavens and a larger perspective.

The hand is often seen as a symbol of wisdom – not intellectual wisdom but wisdom connected to the body and our own individual nature. The hand, suggesting her very own individuality in the center, also suggests her new sense of self – she makes her own individual statement and asserts herself in her very own way. It was already clear that by this time Tammy was becoming more integrated into her ordinary life, having fewer conflicts with friends and

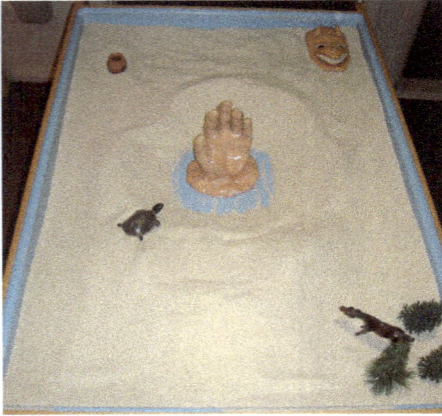

Figure 7.8 Tray 7

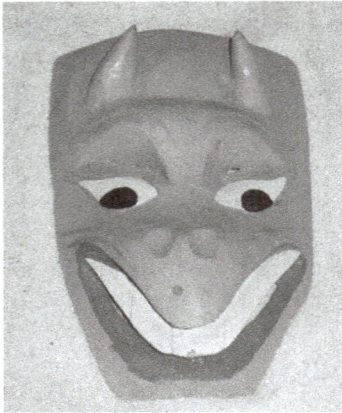

Figure 7.9 Tray 7 detail

seeking out more creative activities, especially in her new pursuit of music. She was making more mature and thoughtful choices, clearly less caught in her old family dynamic.

However, lurking in the background of this otherwise inspirational scene, we see the devil. Just as new possibilities appear for Tammy, the demonic and destructive side of her relationship with the masculine emerges in the image of this horned demon. She had mentioned that the workers in the house had described her father as a "demon." However, the devil can also be thought of a positive aspect of the masculine energy as well as a dangerous aspect of the dark side of the masculine in her. So, it was another reminder of both the fertile and demonic aspects that were latent within her.

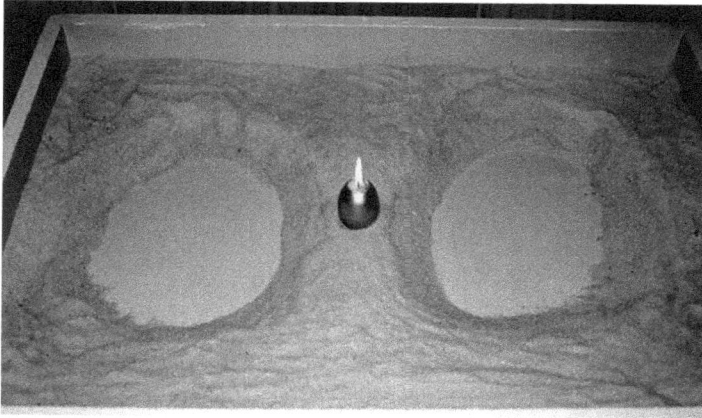

Figure 7.10 Tray 8

Figure 7.10 (Tray 8)

Split but *Centered*: this tray was created about a month after the former tray – a week before Easter. When Tammy came to the session, she brought with her a beautiful golden egg made of wax and said that she wanted to make a tray so she could use the egg in it and then light it so we both could sit together and watch it burn.

She began working in her old style of making two separate circles, a tray reminiscent of many before. However, after she made the circles, she carefully placed the golden egg between the two circles and lit it. She then asked if we could watch the candle together for a while until the session was over and, also, as the candle burned down during the day, would I watch it and the next time we met, tell her how long it took to burn out and what it looked like throughout the day? I felt the specialness of the moment and the extraordinary task that she had asked of me, to essentially think about her for an entire day. I realized she was speaking about the trust that she now had in me. The egg is generally an extremely positive symbol, pointing to the potential creation of new conscious attitudes. Jung said that out of the egg emerges "the liberated soul" – representing new psychic contents and carrying the regeneration of the spirit and the new personality. After her appointment, I did leave my office with the candle and watched it burn down at home.

Figure 7.11 (Tray 9)

In this tray, there is still a slight split, but it is *Bridged*. The two circles now have become hearts with a bridge connecting them. And for the second time, Tammy is able to span the great divide under the gaze of the queen and two peacocks and a green frog watching it all unfold. As she made this tray she said: "today I can take my time making this tray and let it be, and I'm not feeling rushed to hurry up and make up my mind about what to do."

About the frog observing this scene: first and foremost the frog is about transformation, moving through many stages of development – from an egg to a polliwog and then to an adult

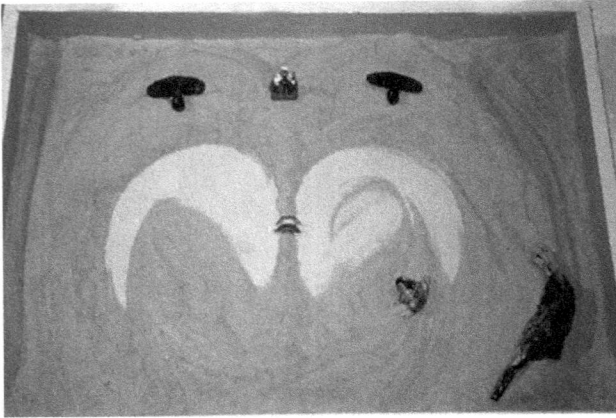

Figure 7.11 Tray 9

frog. Jung speaks to the meaning of the frog in modern dreams as "the animal urge in us all toward life."

In the exact place where Tammy put the fire in the previous tray, there is now a bridge; something was energized, as symbolized by the fire. The energy is now there to bridge her split.

Figure 7.12 Tray 10)

Tammy, again, made this tray in a meditative manner, able to turn off her internal chatter and make more space in both her mind and body for something new to be born under the gaze of one personal mother overlooking the baby Jesus and another more distant and archetypal mother outside the sacred circle.

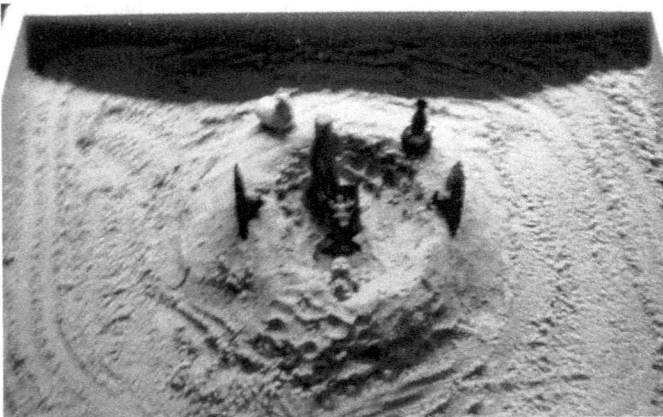

Figure 7.12 Tray 10

However, she did remark, "that baby has only one mother, and one day he'll be able to stand alone." Placing an infant in the tray is often a symbol of unification of the opposites, i.e., a healer, one who makes things whole. I was most encouraged to see this infant, clearly pointing ahead to the possibility of change.

Four healing themes are present in this tray (*Centered, Spiritual, Birthing*, and *Integrated*), and two of the four are quite prominent (2 points). *Integrated* is a new theme for Tammy as she provides a congruent, organized idea that encompasses the tray.

Figure 7.13 (Tray 11)

Only healing themes are present here: *Centered* and *Energized* (greenery). Tammy's ability to actualize her more focused and transformed energy is seen here, as she places a frog (symbol of transformation) in the central circle with the elephant gazing steadily at the frog. Now with enough internal cohesion, Tammy makes one circle with these two animals, while the sacrificial sheep stands over to the left.

After Tammy created this tray, she spoke about how different this tray is from any she had made before and how much gratitude she was feeling for all the changes that were going on in her life.

In her outer life, Tammy was in a new relationship with a male friend and also pursuing a new career involving music. She was finding much satisfaction with both. She was surprised to find that she had new energy to pursue her goals. She had just returned from a trip to her East Coast home and for the first time had been able to set limits with her family by making arrangements beforehand to visit her mom and her nanny separately, therefore avoiding many of the old tensions with them. She was able to speak freely with them about her new life with her male friend and her new interest in music. She was no longer self-conscious and concerned about their judgment of her. She said that it was the least stressful time she could ever remember having with her family.

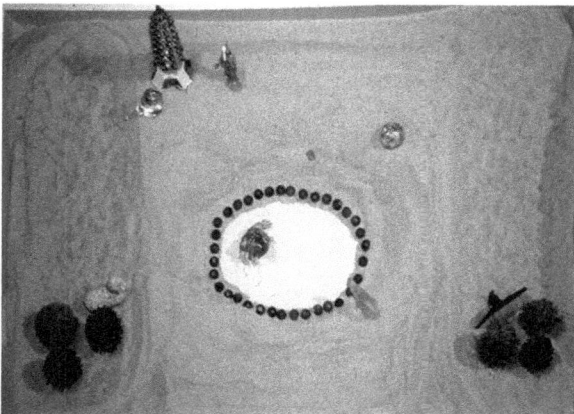

Figure 7.13 Tray 11

Figures 7.14 and 7.15 (Tray 12)

In the middle of this large central space, Tammy places an old-fashioned hurricane lamp to bring new light to an old situation. In the upper right-hand corner on a tiny mountain, she puts a single mother holding a baby. Nearby, another woman stands as an observer, close by but not interrupting the mother and baby. Overlooking this scene she places two more large lamps, bringing light to the scene.

A new theme is seen here: *Nurturing*. In the sand picture, the mother is supporting the baby, suggesting a supportive family group. However, the round lake is the most prominent theme in this tray – the theme of *Centered*. In addition, *Energy* is also seen with the green trees.

She said as she finished the tray, "this place in me feels so good, so good to be here finally."

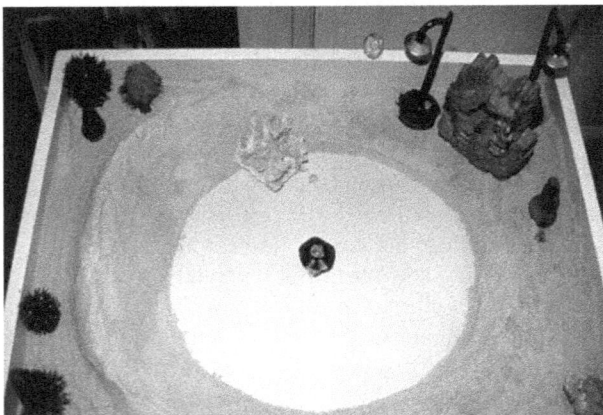

Figure 7.14 Tray 12

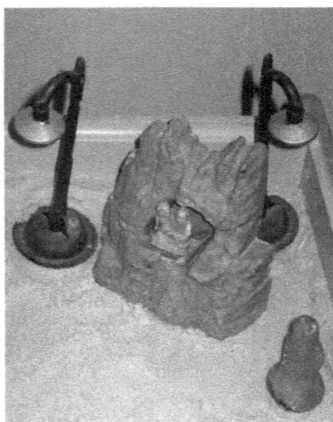

Figure 7.15 Tray 12 detail

Figures 7.16 and 7.17 (Tray 13)

This was a powerful moment when Tammy smoothed the sand and then placed both of her hands in the center of the tray, pressing them hard, making sure she had made a clear impression in the sand. As Tammy made the hand prints in the tray, she began to cry, and she spoke of her gratitude for the huge changes that had taken place in these years of therapy.

She was feeling moved by the same age-old energy that has moved men and woman since time began – to put their hand prints wherever they went to make their own individual mark. Earlier Tammy placed a hand in the middle of Tray 7. Now she uses her own hands to make her personal statement.

There are two themes in this tray: *Centered* and *Energized* (moving her hands in a circle).

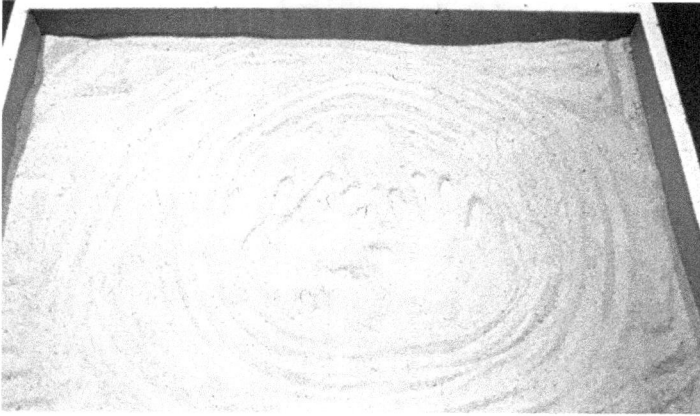

Figure 7.16 Tray 13

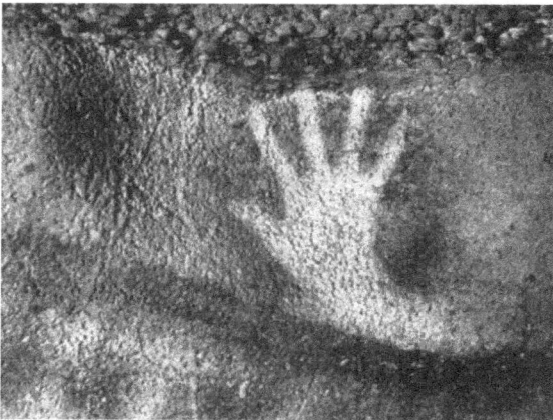

Figure 7.17 Ancient hand print on a cave wall

Figures 7.18 and 7.19 (Tray 14)

In this tray, only healing themes are evident, particularly the healing themes of *Bridging*, *Centered*, and *Spiritual*.

When she finished making this scene, Tammy said, "I just love this tray; it's so beautiful. I know about this place in me now and it feels so good there."

In this tray, a woman is carrying a baby. She crosses over a bridge toward the mountain, leading to the jade tree and the harp on the top. The harp possibly refers to her new interest in her own feelings, as well as a newly discovered interest in music. It is a place of perspective and objectivity.

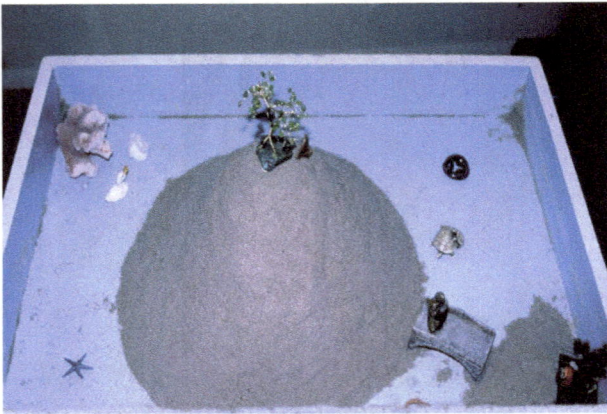

Figure 7.18 Tray 14

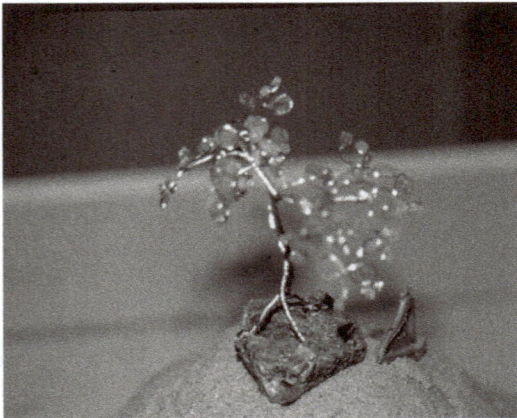

Figure 7.19 Tray 14 detail

Figures 7.20 and 7.21 (Tray 15)

Tammy's final tray was created shortly before she terminated treatment. In a peaceful set-
ting, with a single mother and child over to the right, she creates one large circle containing a
mirror, a starfish, and a glass orb. Overlooking it all, she places a scale balancing two golden
circles.

Tammy has now found a place that can finally balance between the two pulls that have
plagued her for so long, and she now has a sense of her own self, as well as a feeling of equi-
librium. This final tray is a *Centered* and *Integrated* scene and yet it still possesses *Energy*.

The next seven figures illustrate the evolution (development) of themes in the series of
trays just discussed:

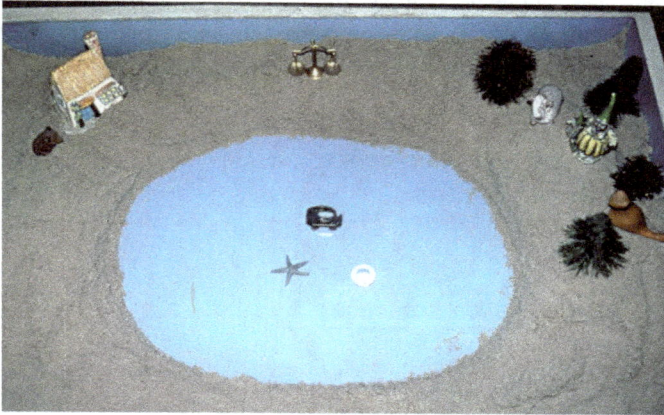

Figure 7.20 Tray 15

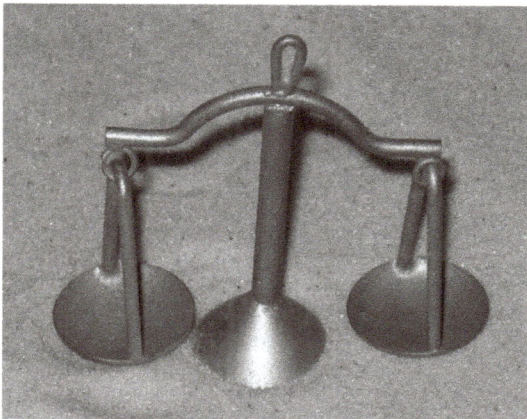

Figure 7.21 Tray 15 detail

- **Figure 7.22** shows that Trays 1, 2, and 3 are all split, but the split becomes smaller, less prominent, and changed in positive ways
- **Figure 7.23** demonstrates that in Trays 4, 5, and 8 the split become even less prominent and changed in positive ways
- **Figure 7.24** demonstrates that in Trays 2, 7, and 8 centering becomes more prominent and enriched
- **Figure 7.25** shows that centering in Tray 12 is larger when compared with Trays 10 and 11 and other previous centered trays
- **Figure 7.26** shows that Tray 13 is creative, energetic, and personal; Tray 14 is prominent and enlarged; and Tray 15 is centered and more prominent and realistic. Realism is important. Dora Kalff said that final trays often show regular life in more realistic trays
- **Figure 7.27** is a table summarizing the major themes in each of the 15 trays
- **Figure 7.28** presents the same summary in a bar graph in which the red bars (in front) represent the extent of wounding themes and the green bars (in back) represent the extent

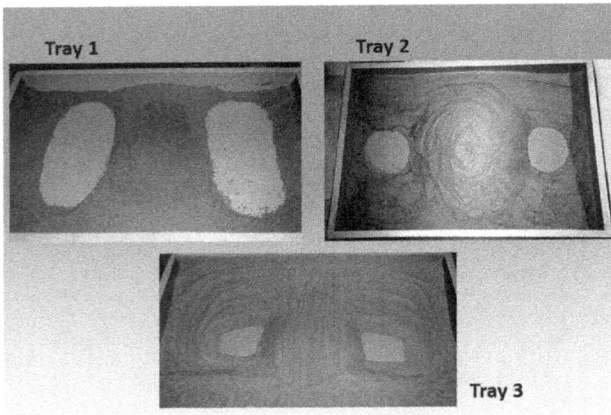

Figure 7.22 Comparison of Trays 1, 2, 3

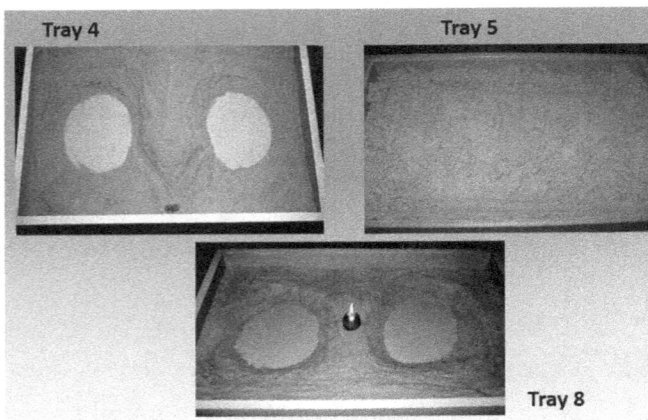

Figure 7.23 Comparison of Trays 4, 5, 8

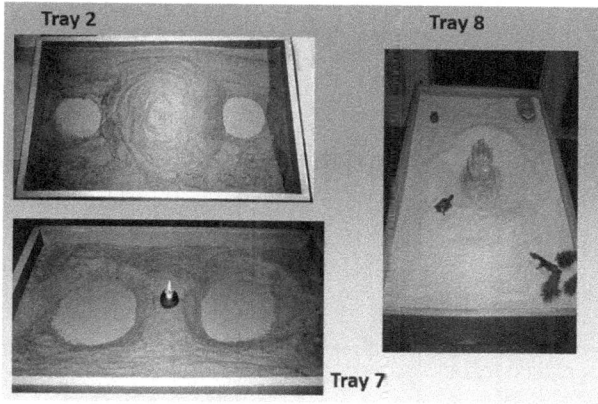

Figure 7.24 Comparison of Trays 2, 7, 8

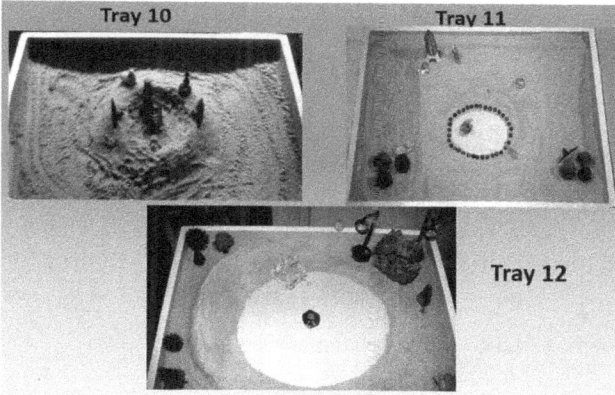

Figure 7.25 Comparison of Trays 10, 11, 12

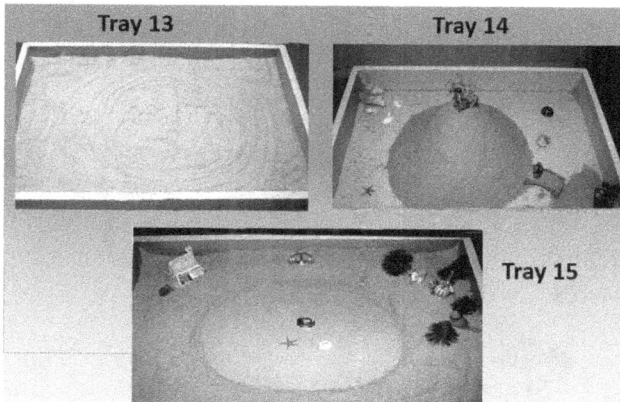

Figure 7.26 Comparison of Trays 13, 14, 15

Sandplay Themes Expressed in the Transformation Process
Case of Tammy
X = Present
XX = Prominent

TRAY #	CHAOTIC	EMPTY	SPLIT	CONFINED	NEGLECTED	HIDDEN	PRONE	INJURED	THREATENED	HINDERED	BRIDGED	JOURNEY	ENERGIZED	DEEPENED	BIRTHING	NURTURING	CHANGED	SPIRITUAL	CENTERED	INTEGRATED
	Wounding Themes										Healing Themes									
1		XX	XX																	
2		X	XX														XX			I
3			XX										X						X	
4			XX														X			
5	XX		X																	
6		XX																		
7													X						XX	
8			XX																X	
9											XX									
10																X		XX	XX	X
11													X						XX	
12													X				X		XX	
13													XX						XX	
14											XX							XX	X	
15													X						XX	XX

Figure 7.27 Table summarizing themes in Tammy's trays

Sandplay Themes in the Transformation Process
Case of Tammy
Red = Wounding   Green = Healing

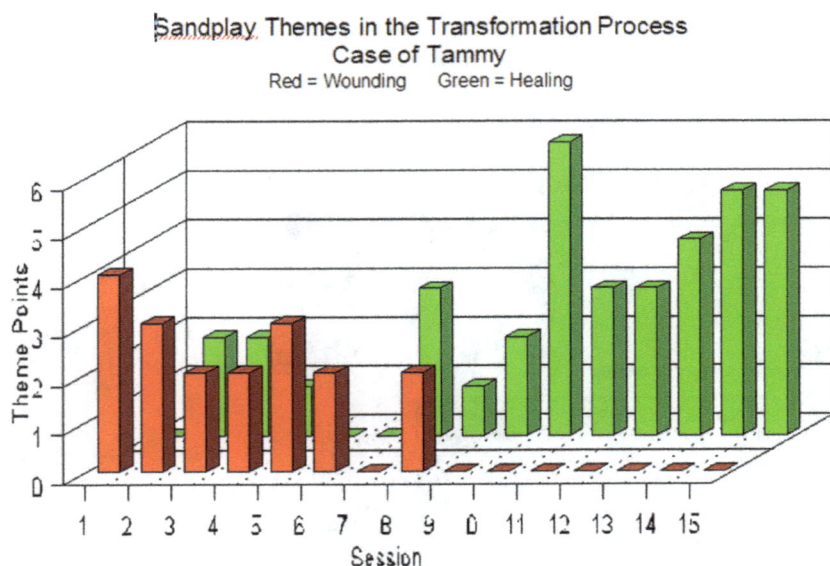

Figure 7.28 Bar graph summarizing themes in Tammy's trays

of healing themes. One can observe the steady disappearance of wounding themes and the growth of healing themes

Some practical considerations

- How do we introduce and use sandplay in a practice (for those new to this modality)?
- How do we ultimately use all this information about symbols and themes in our clinical work?
- How do we encourage and support our own clients in using and experiencing the miniatures, these symbols on our shelves, and then how do we understand what themes are emerging from their sand creations?
- How do we clinicians maintain and hold on to a metaphorical attitude as we follow the meandering symbolic process in clients' sandplays in order to better identify these themes of wounding and healing that follow this often mysterious process?

Introducing and using sandplay

1. It is necessary to have a wide variety of miniatures available, e.g., people, animals, buildings, fences, bridges, vegetation, vehicles, marbles, etc.
2. The miniatures should be arranged on shelves for easy recognition and access
3. It is an advantage to have two trays, one dry and one wet. The trays should be prepared for the client ahead of time. Be sure there are no hidden objects left in the sand from a previous client. Level the sand in both trays. Have water accessible nearby in case the client feels the need to use more
4. When introducing the client to the sand trays, first observe if he/she shows any interest in the sand. Notice which clients gravitate to it and which ones pull away and are uninterested in it
5. If a client shows an interest, invite him/her "to make a picture in the sand"
6. Suggest that your client feel the sand in both trays (to become connected to Mother Earth). Briefly and simply show him/her the shelves and baskets of items and then step back and let the process evolve
7. Create a free and protected space for the client. Be a supportive, neutral, and attentive presence. Accept the expression as it evolves with no comment about what or how items are being used
8. Often the therapist sits a little behind the client and takes notes on the order of the miniatures placed in the tray and their movement, client comments, and therapist's thoughts (Some therapists draw a picture of the sand picture for their notes)
9. Usually clients will know intuitively when they are finished. They will often stand back from the tray and announce, "I'm done"
10. Ask the client if he/she would like to say anything about the picture. Sometimes the client will begin to talk about certain items or themes. These associations amplify the experience for both client and therapist
11. Usually the therapist does not discuss the sand pictures in much depth with the client at this time, as moving too soon to a cognitive level can hinder the evolving nonverbal process. However, listening attentively and noting a client's associations and stories, if forthcoming, are all part of the experience
12. After the client has left, a photograph of the tray should be taken

13. After the sandplay process has been completed and the time feels right to the therapist and client, the process can be reviewed together by viewing the photographs of the client's sandplay scenes

How themes help therapists

Most sandplay therapists are process oriented, i.e., they follow the changes in their clients' sandplay trays over time. However, many sandplay therapists have been more inclined to look at the symbolic content of each tray, rather than the connections between the symbols from one tray to another. We have found it helpful to follow the evolving movement of the psyche in the trays using the set of process themes presented in this chapter to identify and track the archetypal themes that emerge in the sandplay creations. A sandplay theme is an intrinsic organization within the psyche.

Such changes as seen here in Tammy's trays evolve over time. Following archetypal themes in the sandplay process assists in understanding the language of the client's unconscious. As we view the progression of themes in our clients' trays, we can gain a sense of what is happening in the core of the client's psyche, as well as monitoring psychological changes and determining how the client is responding to therapy.

Chapter 8

Age and gender issues

As we worked with sandplay, we realized not all our adult clients made trays that looked like typical adult trays. Upon reflection, many of them were indistinguishable from trays that children make. We began to realize that these younger looking trays were alerting us to unresolved issues and traumas resulting from earlier experiences in these clients' lives. These issues were still alive in the unconscious and were revealed in trays.

This chapter presents and discusses sandplay creations of females and males at various ages and is organized to help identify which features in trays are related to age, which to gender, and which to the uniqueness of the individual psyche, as well as to determine what is age-appropriate, and what is not and thus may suggest a problem.

The following discussion of age and gender effects is organized around the five sandplay categories used in the research by Ruth Bowyer Pickford (1956):

1. The use of space
2. Expression of aggression
3. Control in and coherence of the tray
4. Use of the sand
5. Contents of the tray

Dr. Bowyer Pickford (her research and writing was under the name "Bowyer") was a researcher and colleague of Margaret Lowenfeld. In the 1950s, she made major contributions to the sandplay literature by studying the sand trays of 50 children and 26 adults between the ages of two and 50 to create developmental norms. The sand trays were created by "normal" individuals who were not in therapy. Bowyer's five categories and developmental norms are illustrated with sand trays from our practices. Also included are examples of trays from clients with prior wounding issues.

Bowyer's norms are a primary resource for the influence of age on sandplay creations. This chapter also includes and compares what other researchers have now added with regard to influence of age as well as gender. The researchers include Kamp and Kessler (1970) and Kamp, Ambrosius and Zwaan (1986). The latter study examined how chronological age and mental health of children affect the way miniatures are organized in the tray. Also included is information from a large study by Linn Jones (1986). She examined age differences in the sand tray for children between 11 months and 18 years to determine if the differences were consistent with Piaget's theories. She also researched the effect gender has on sand tray creations. Jones' study supports the belief of both Piaget and Jung that a central organizing principle determines the development of the human psyche.

In examining the following sand play pictures, it becomes evident that various stages of archetypal development weave in and out of the trays. In each case there is either age-appropriate development or development disrupted by some kind of wounding at a crucial stage. Both categories are illustrated in child, teenage, and adult trays. For example, if an adult experienced wounding at age seven, some aspects of his/her trays may look somewhat like that of a seven-year-old.

In examining pictures of the following trays, it can be useful to turn one eye inward and notice which scenes – which motifs – in the trays reach out and resonate with you personally, perhaps as one might do when listening to a dream. Noting the places of personal resonance in a sandplay can become a particularly rich source of information and can provide insight that the intellect cannot. Jung (1969) wrote in 1927, "Often the hands know how to solve a riddle with which the intellect has wrestled in vain."

Bowyer's first category: The use of space

The first category Bowyer created was the area of the tray used. She found that, with increasing age, a greater and greater area of the tray is used and a better sense of control and coherence is displayed. Older children use more of the tray and show a firmer sense of boundaries.

The following are examples of trays from children as well as adult trays that look about the same as those of the children. The first two trays, created by very young children, show what is typical of two, three, and four-year-olds as they work in a sandplay environment. These trays are dramatically different from trays of older children and adults that follow. Bowyer's research demonstrates that young children typically use only a small section of the tray; essentially the rest of the tray is ignored and sand may even be spilled over the sides of the tray. Her research also reveals that boundaries and outer reality are disregarded, and heaps of toys are often thrown or flung into the tray. By the age of six and beyond, children usually begin to use the space out to all four sides of the tray, while the clinical population sometimes uses only a portion of the tray.

Figure 8.1

This first tray was created by a two-and-a-half-year-old girl who was unexpectedly brought to her mother's therapy session. The child went immediately over to the tray, picked up a watering can close to the tray, and watered only a small portion of the tray. An older child with more hand-eye coordination would most probably have moistened more of the tray and have done so with more focus. This particular child then tipped over the watering can and left it there, half in and half out the tray, indicating a lack of boundaries. This tray is typical and normal for children in her very young age group.

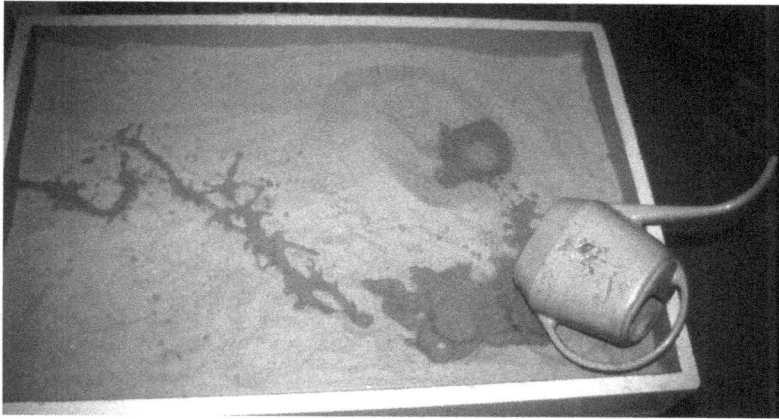

Figure 8.1 Tray of a two-and-a-half-year-old girl

Figure 8.2

This tray – containing cars, trucks, and people all heaped together in the center – was created by a four-year-old boy. He selected the toys he liked, carried them over to the tray, and dumped them in. He did this several times. There is noticeable chaos, and numerous objects are used in a freely disorganized fashion; however, it is a little more complex than Figure 8.1. All his objects remain inside the tray, boundaries are more recognized, and more of the tray has been used than in the previous one, created by a younger child. This type of chaotic tray is seen regularly in trays of four-year-olds.

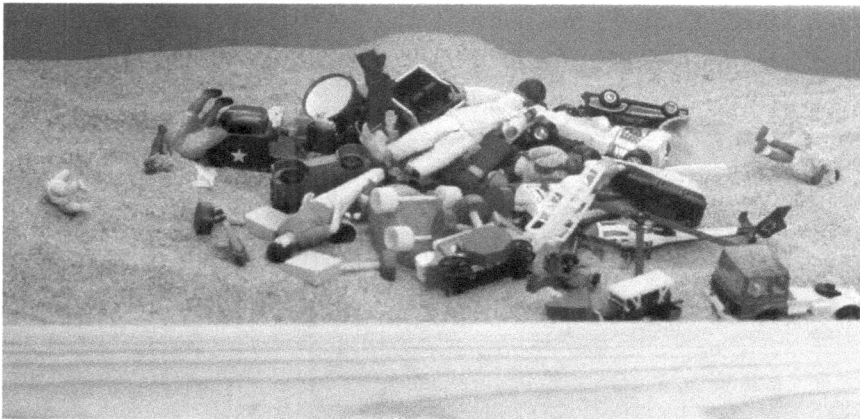

Figure 8.2 Tray of a four-year-old boy

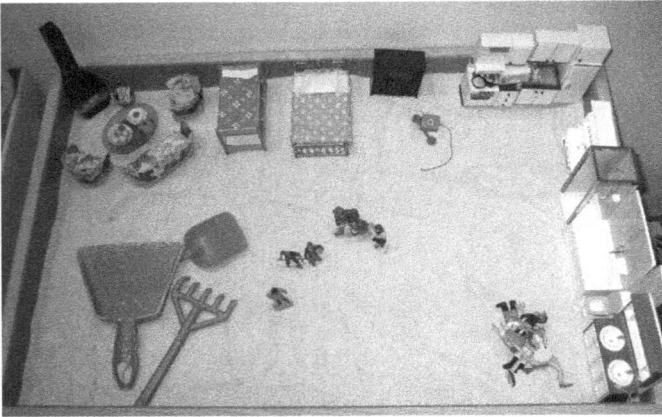

Figure 8.3 Tray of an eight-year-old girl

Figure 8.3

This creation, by an eight-year-old girl, uses the entire tray, in contrast to the two previous trays. This tray illustrates how an older child utilizes the space. This realistic scene is also illustrative of the results from Kamp and Kessler's (1970) work, researching children six to nine years old. They found that: (a) children's organization of miniatures within the tray becomes more realistic as they get older, and (b) the trays of more intelligent children were more realistic than those of other same-aged children.

Figure 8.4

Now – a big developmental jump to a sandplay of a 40-year-old man who was in an enraged and regressed state. This man had recently been accused of acting inappropriately with a customer at work. He felt misunderstood and wrongly accused. This situation evoked childhood

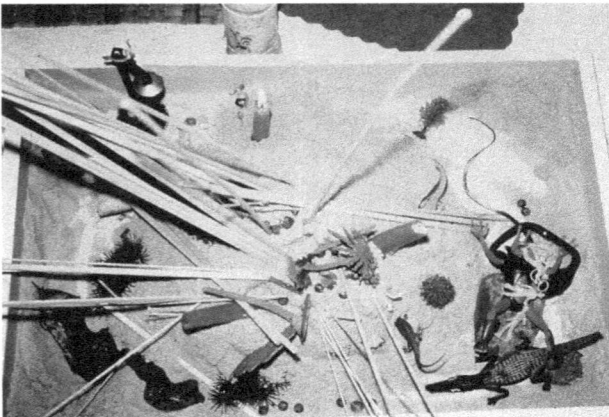

Figure 8.4 Tray of a 40-year-old man

feelings and memories of having been misunderstood and wounded, growing up in a chaotic, cult-like religious environment. His family moved into this community when he was about four years old. Notice how he uses the space. His tray is similar a young child's chaotic tray, and dramatically illustrates the rage and chaos he was feeling. His tray is a powerful communication about the overwhelming feelings experienced by him as a child under the age of five. Here, it appears that these feelings are still alive for him.

Figure 8.5

A 42-year-old woman uses only a small portion of this tray. She was the oldest of seven children, now married to a professional pianist. She expressed the despair and lack of identity she was feeling in her life, and conveyed this in a very young manner. As the oldest child in her family of origin, she had learned to devote herself to helping and serving others, but she felt stuck in this pattern and, by this time, these feelings had become an obstacle to her development. This tray, depicting a solitary piano (her husband's instrument), communicated the barren state that living for and serving others had ultimately created for her.

A tray with only one miniature is quite unusual for adults. Usually, adult trays are complex with many miniatures. Several studies support this observation. Jones (1986) found that sand worlds become more structurally complex with age. Kamp, Ambrosius, and Zwaan (1986) found significant differences between disturbed and normal children with regard to their use of miniatures in the tray. Normal children's trays appeared richer, fuller, and less blocked, while disturbed children's trays were less well defined and seemed incomplete. Disturbed adults exhibited a similar pattern with trays that appeared chaotic, less defined, and/or empty, such as these last two adult trays.

In summary, the following three features characterize the use of space in young children's trays: (a) only a small portion of the tray is used; (b) there is a lack of boundaries; and/or (c)

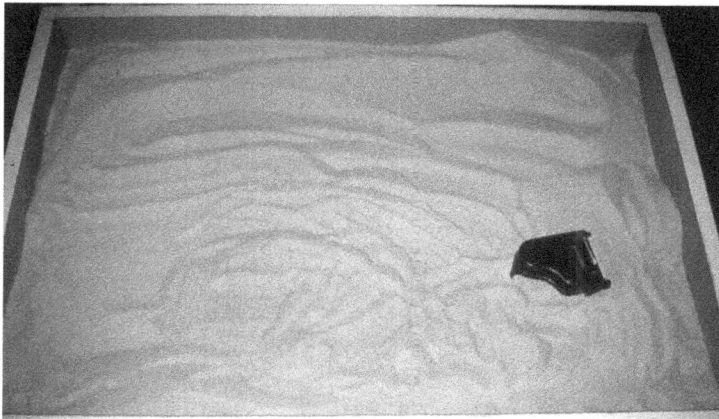

Figure 8.5 Tray of a 42-year-old woman

figures often tend to be heaped in the tray. These features also appear in adult trays when individuals are severely regressed or psychologically undeveloped.

Figure 8.6

Four and five-year-olds seem to be in transition, with some children using a small portion of the tray and others placing toys at intervals throughout the tray. This picture was created by a five-year-old boy. At first glance it looks very young, with only two miniatures at the back of the tray, a boat and an airplane. However, note the marks in the sand: he moved the boat around in the sand, staying within the margins of the tray. This is a good example of a transition tray – use of only a few miniatures but staying within the boundaries and being aware of the entire tray – in this case by moving the boat around in the sand.

The symbolism of the two miniatures he used is important in understanding his tray. His mother died from a brain tumor when he was three-and-a-half years old. When he first came to therapy, he was in mourning, acting out and refusing to do anything at school. Boats are often used by children to suggest the mother; notice how far it is from where he is standing. He took the airplane and crashed it beside the boat. Probably the airplane represents him; he was very angry and felt lost without her. Remember that the tray is a picture of the psyche. When he moved the boat all over the tray, it may have been to show that his mother had made a large imprint on his psyche. Later in therapy, we talked about his belief that his mother was in heaven watching him. After our discussion of his mother watching over him, movement was made in his accepting her death and his being able to carry her with him – inside of himself.

Another note about this tray. When he moved the boat around the tray and crashed the plane into the sand – that was movement of miniatures in play. This is what many sandplay therapists call a dynamic picture or a dynamic sandplay. Children at eight years or younger

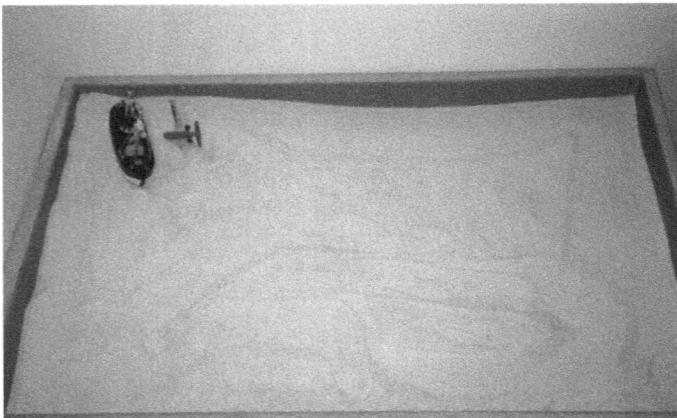

Figure 8.6 Tray of a five-year-old boy

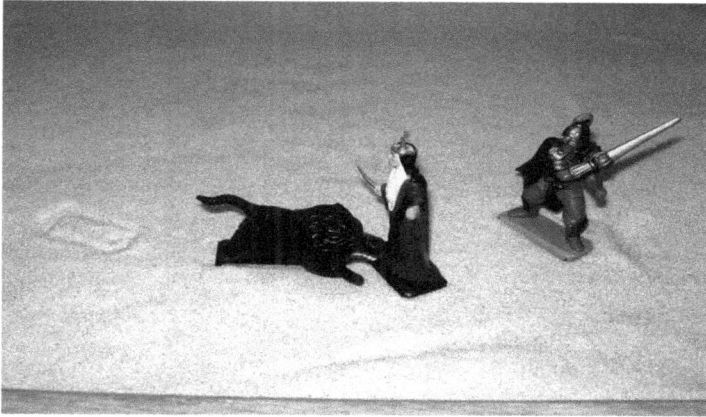

Figure 8.7 Tray of a 46-year-old woman

often make dynamic pictures; however, after about age eight, children and adults almost always create stationary pictures (the miniatures are placed as if they are painting a picture rather than playing with them or moving them around). This may be because, in their minds, they are showing movement without moving the figures. If an adult or a child over eight years of age creates a dynamic picture, it is considered diagnostically significant, suggesting that there may be a reason for this person to craft a younger tray – perhaps a childhood trauma.

Figure 8.7

This tray was made by a 46-year-old woman. It contains only three miniatures: a ferocious dog, a queen holding a knife, and a gladiator with a sword. The ferocious dog was placed first, followed by the others. The client then stood beside the tray and stared at it for about five minutes. Dramatically, she moved the dog toward the queen and had it bite the queen. This is a dynamic picture with few miniatures and typically very young. This was the only sandplay picture this client made, although she was in therapy for three years. In my long experience as a therapist, she was the most abused client I have ever seen. She was physically and sexually abused by both parents. The family lived in a cult, and she was also abused by cult members from birth through her teen years.

Figure 8.8

This tray illustrates how the entire space is used when there has been a significant healing experience in therapy. An image such as this one is very often an end product of therapy. A 37-year-old woman created this tray toward the end of her treatment. The feeling of centeredness, liveliness, a greater connection to her own spirituality, and the strong statement of increased consciousness (as symbolized by the lighted candles and feathers), clearly communicate her strong sense of self.

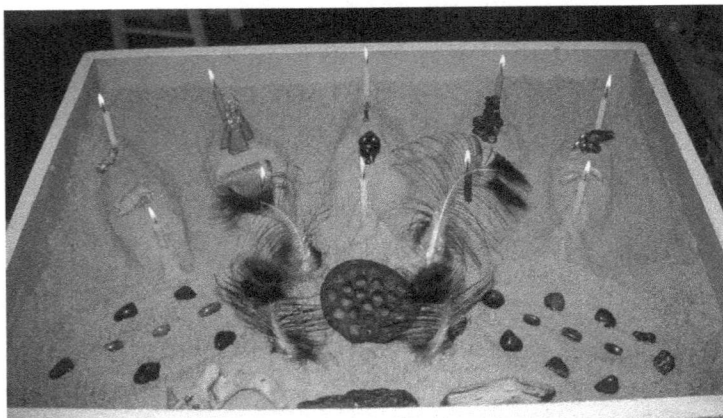

Figure 8.8 Tray of a 37-year-old woman

Expression of aggression

Bowyer's second category deals with how the expression of aggression changes as normal development unfolds. She observed that two-to-three-year-olds often poke, fling, or bury miniatures, while four-to-six-year-olds use dramatic activity in moving the toys around in the tray, often making noises and speaking for the miniatures they are using.

One of her very interesting findings was that aggression was often found in the trays of normal children and adults. Therefore, it appears that aggression in the tray is not diagnostically significant; aggression does not differentiate normal children from those who have severe problems.

However, Bowyer did find that aggression is expressed differently depending on the age. She found that normal two-to-three-year-olds most often poked, flung, or buried miniatures. Four-to-six-year-olds particularly use dramatic activity by moving the toys around in the tray. They often had their miniatures fight with each other, and the children even made noises and spoke for the miniatures they were using. Dynamic trays, fighting miniatures, as well as moving and making noises for the miniatures are quite typical for children eight or younger. The following tray is an example.

Figure 8.9

This creation, depicting two monsters eating a mother and father, was made by a five-year-old boy as he made growling noises and moved the figures about. Without being aware of developmental norms, one might conclude that this is a very disturbed child instead of realizing his behavior is quite typical and appropriate for his age group. However, the symbolism of eating the mother and father did reflect this child's anger at his parents being in a very conflictual divorce, and each parent trying to win him over to his/her side.

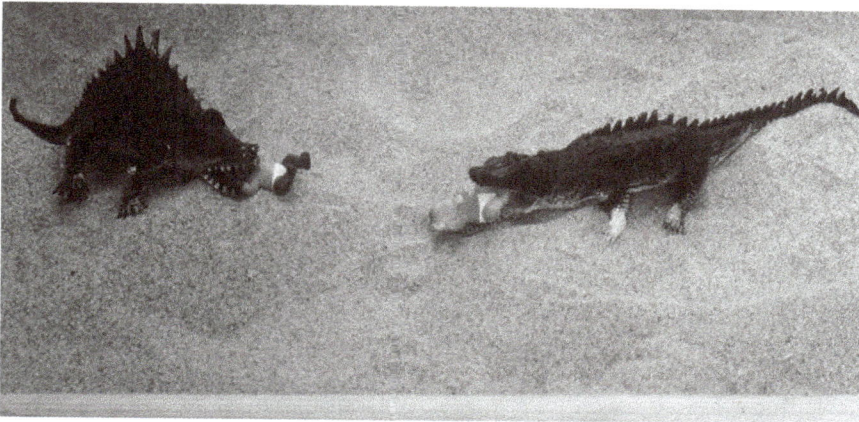

Figure 8.9 Tray of a five-year-old boy

Figure 8.10

The parents of this seven-year-old boy had divorced when he was two years old. He used the miniatures and sand to create two clearly delineated camps. This picture conveys his own anger, as well as his parents' divisiveness. Two armies are actively shooting at each other while he rides in a canoe in the middle of the tray, attempting to go back and forth between the two camps. As he was creating this tray and moving the canoe back and forth making shooting sounds, he said, "This is how it feels to come home to my mom's house after I've been with my dad all weekend long. The fighting just never stops."

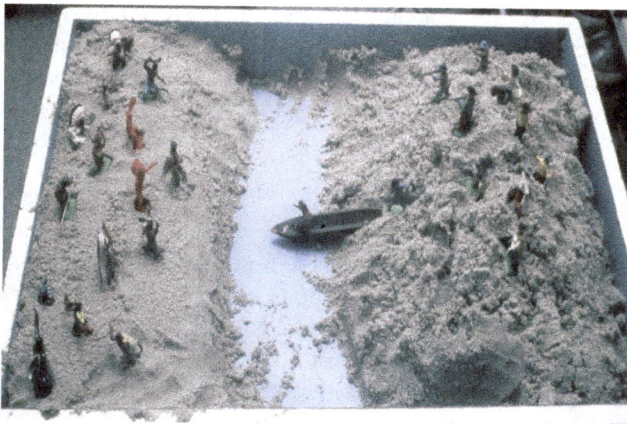

Figure 8.10 Tray of a seven-year-old boy

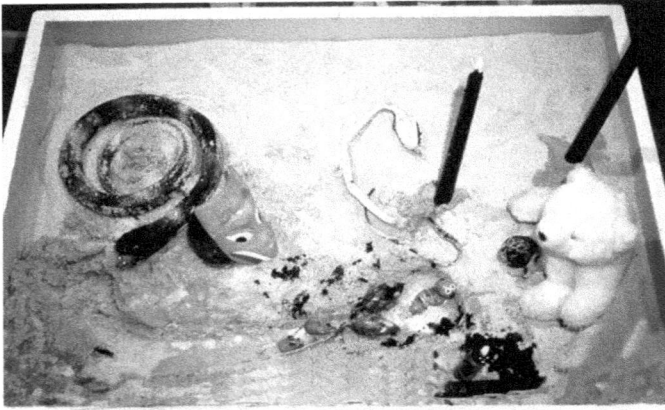

Figure 8.11 Tray of a 40-year-old woman

Figure 8.11

This tray, which demonstrates a young stage of aggression, illustrates how early wounding can be seen in a tray. It was created by a 40-year-old unmarried woman who had come to treatment in great distress after impulsively having an abortion. She had lost what she now believed was her last chance to have her own baby. She told me that her mother had talked her into it. She was now overwrought, full of remorse, and suffering from feelings of loss about the abortion. She felt she had been tricked by her mother once again. As she made the tray, she repeatedly thrust the snake forward as if it were biting at the mask and spoke about how she had always been forced to act in ways her mother dictated. She felt consumed with rage at her mother. Perhaps the snake depicts her mother's aggression and/or her own anger.

From about eight years old, and certainly by twelve years of age through adulthood, moving objects around in the tray subsides. Clients seem to be more consciously aware of their aggressive feelings and appear content to depict these feelings in the tray without needing to move figures, interact with them, or make sounds for the miniatures. At eight years old, the frontal lobes start to develop, which coincides with the emergence of an objective and observing ego. At 12, qualitative differences happen in the frontal lobes, and the child becomes even more aware. However, it is not until around 25 years old that the frontal lobes fully mature.

Control in and coherence of the tray

In early developmental stages, little or no control is shown by two-to-four-year-olds; their trays are typically chaotic, undifferentiated, and disorganized. Bowyer (1956) found that control tends to expand from five to ten years of age, for example, as evidenced by an increased use of fencing. Ten years is the peak age for using fences and other literal structures of control. After 11 years, there is less use of literal controls and more use of symbolic controls. After 11 years, issues of control are expressed more often by the use of topological features, such as mountains and streams, to unify the scene in the tray.

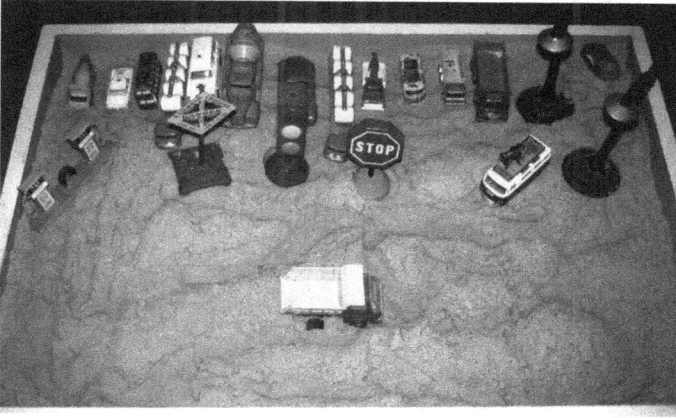

Figure 8.12 Tray of a nine-year-old boy

Figure 8.12

This nine-year-old boy had a violent history of acting out toward his two older siblings. In this tray, he shows the development of the use of space, his ability to tell his story about these cars that had to stop, as well as his use of literal stop signs to control the cars.

Figure 8.13

This ten-year-old girl's tray demonstrates how fencing is often used by children around ten years old, the peak age for fencing. Here, the high level of sexual energies, as symbolized by the horses, is safely differentiated from the domestic, more feminine energies – appropriate at this prepubescent age.

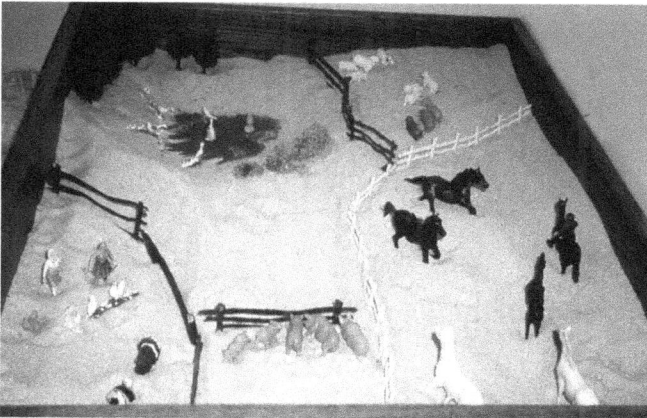

Figure 8.13 Tray of a ten-year-old girl

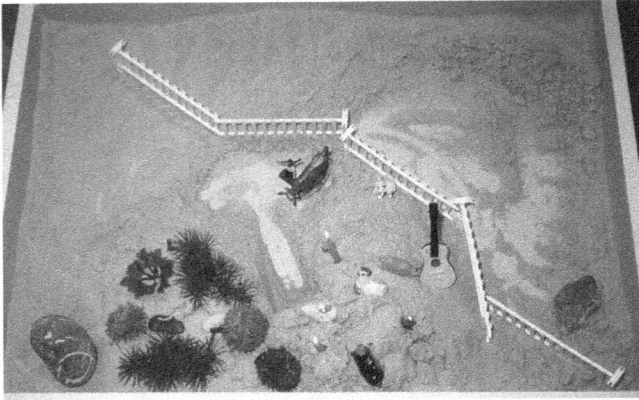

Figure 8.14 Tray of a 29-year-old man

Figure 8.14

This tray demonstrates another use of fencing – this time by a 29-year-old man who felt betrayed in a love affair. The woman with whom he had planned a life together had left him for another man. When he was 11, his mother had died suddenly. The upper area of devastation, portraying his wounding, is literally fenced off, much like an 11-year-old would do. However, it was positive to see that growth was possible even in his current depressed state. I was hopeful that future therapeutic work would help him manifest these potentials for a new life.

Figures 8.15 and 8.16

Adults use more symbolic controls in sandplay than younger individuals. This 47-year-old woman who was feeling abandoned because her last child had just left for college poignantly displays symbolic control. When she was a child, her father left home when her mother was

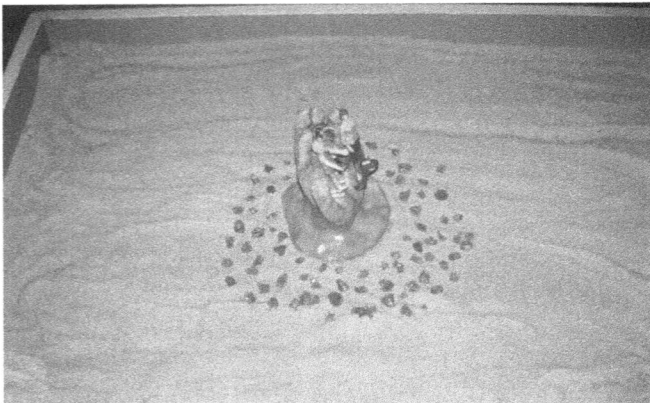

Figure 8.15 Tray of a 47-year-old woman

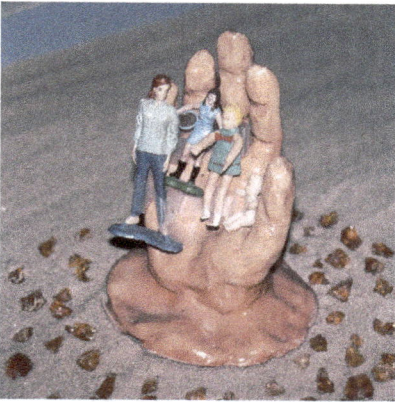

Figure 8.16 Tray of a 47-year-old woman, detail

pregnant with her to fight in the Second World War and didn't return until she was five. Her parents divorced two years after he returned. This woman had never recovered from her early and prolonged yearning to be part of an intact family. Now, decades later, with her last child departing, these feelings, depicted in the hand attempting to hold together her diminishing family, were becoming overwhelming. The central scene, with three girls and a baby in the hand, is made more dramatic by the circles of gem stones.

Use of the sand

It is very interesting to observe the many different ways both children and adults use the sand. Bowyer (1956) noted that young children use sand for pouring, pushing, and burying. After age seven, the constructive use of sand for creating roads, waterways, buildings, and paths appears to depend on individual personality traits more than on age differences. She found that the constructive use of sand to enlarge or restructure the tray indicates an ability to use inner resources creatively and symbolically to change one's own world. She also found that the constructive use of sand suggested average or above-average intelligence.

Figure 8.17

This tray was created by a nine-year-old boy, whose mother had died when he was three. His story that accompanied this tray was about how the boats were trying over and over to get to a safe harbor. His use of sand to construct a safe harbor showed a high level of creativity and healing potential.

Figure 8.18

This 11-year-old boy's sand structure – adorned with shells, rocks, and the American flag – was a celebratory tray. At long last, he had just been accepted onto a Little League baseball

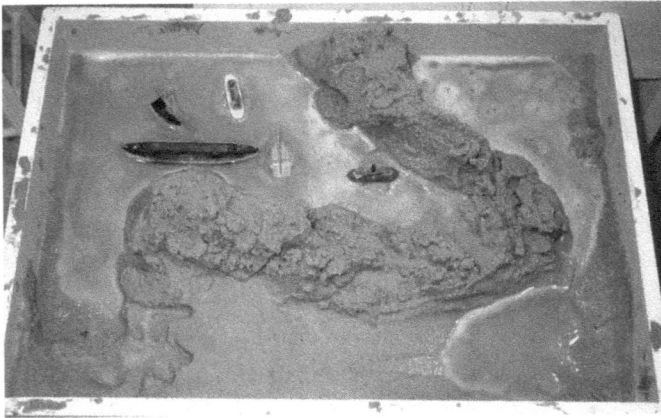

Figure 8.17 Tray of a nine-year-old boy

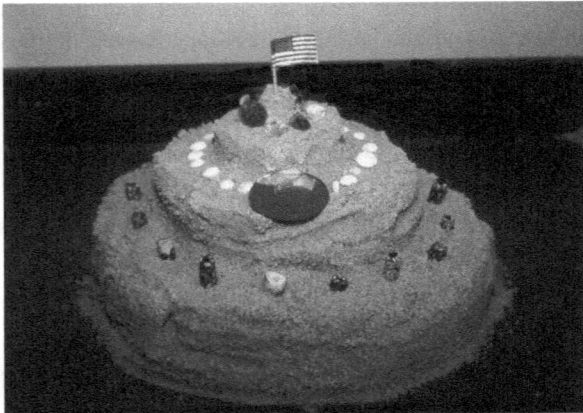

Figure 8.18 Tray of an 11-year-old boy

team. What an effort this tray took for him to construct, and what pleasure he took in viewing it when it was finished. In this achievement, the Self certainly had been constellated.

Figure 8.19

This is a sand construction by a 39-year-old woman, a university administrator, who had just had a professional paper accepted for publication in a prestigious journal. To her, it felt like a culmination of her inner and outer work. The similarity of this tray with that of the previous

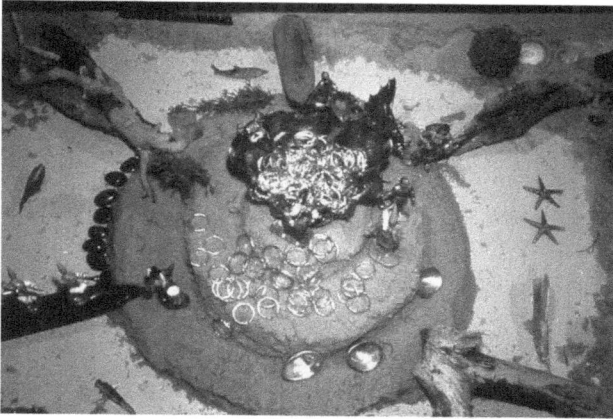

Figure 8.19 Tray of a 39-year-old woman

11-year-old boy's is striking; both trays have used the sand to suggest that the Self has been touched in a profound and deep way.

Figure 8.20

The use of sand in this tray was particularly touching. This 30-year-old woman had been told by her gynecologist that she might never become pregnant due to a physical deformity. Her creative use of the sand, as well as her depiction of her grief with the little rocks, suggests that she is attempting to take in this sad fate.

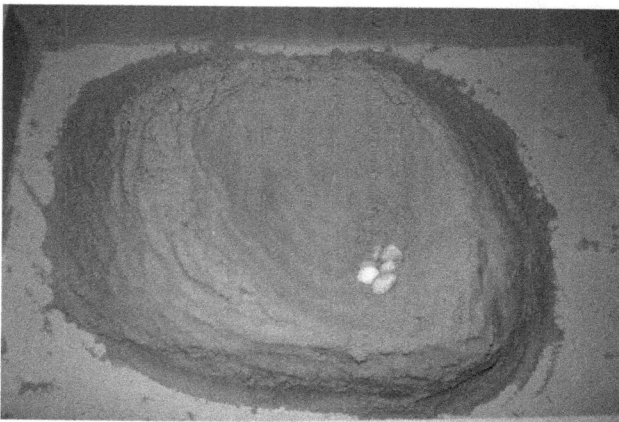

Figure 8.20 Tray of a 30-year-old woman

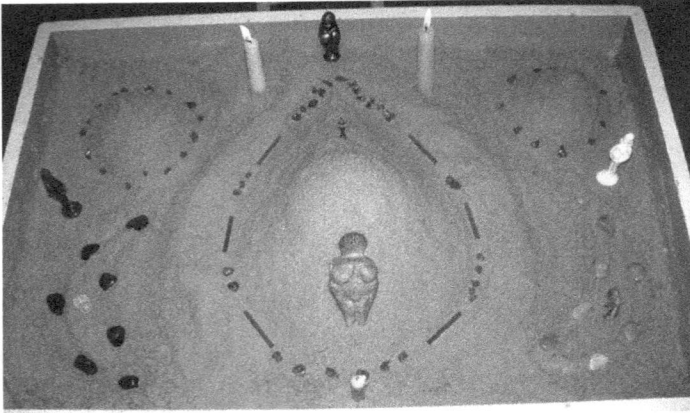

Figure 8.21 Tray of the same 30-year-old woman

Figure 8.21

Six months later she created this tray, and two weeks later she learned that she was pregnant.

Figure 8.22

This tray was made six weeks before the birth of her child. The primitive goddess figure stands upright, overlooking the scene, while the human infant now stands between two breast-like mounds.

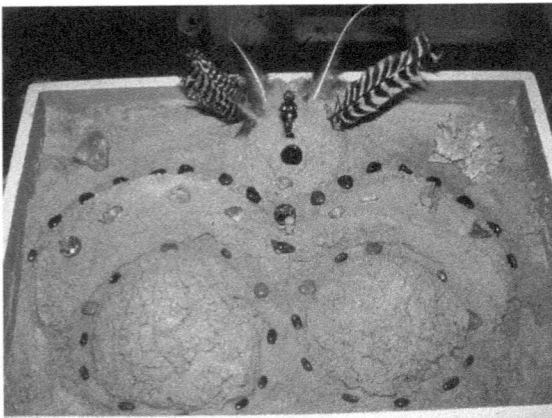

Figure 8.22 Tray of same 30 year old woman

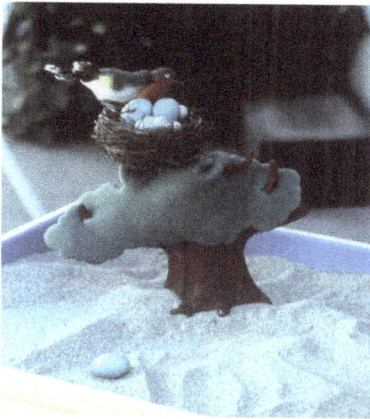

Figure 8.23 Tray of a six-year-old girl

Contents of the tray

Bowyer's fifth and last category refers to the contents of the tray. She found that, with increasing age, realism increases, miniatures are more integrated, and a time perspective is often included. Trays of children of the same age show great similarities under eight years of age, but, after about eight years of age, individual differences in trays begin to emerge and trays are highly individualized, so developmental norms do not fit as clearly.

Figure 8.23

The content and story told about this sandplay created by a six-year-old girl shows both realism and fantasy, although not as clearly as those done by older children. Her older sister had died when this girl was a year-and-a-half old. She placed the nest on top of the tree and then she took one of the eggs and dropped it on the sand, saying, "The mommy bird is looking for her egg. She can't take care of her other eggs because she just keeps looking for her lost egg."

Figure 8.24

This realistic tray of a 12-year-old boy depicts a baseball team playing on a diamond, a mandala, with cavemen looking on (suggesting old issues are off to one side). The boy said, "The cavemen stand on the side as the game is coming to a close. They remember how these guys never even used to be able to throw a ball." This tray was created just as this boy's therapy was terminating. When he began therapy he had been physically immature and frightened of entering into the world, as well as into the game of life. Here he is a true participant in life, all played out on a diamond, a unifying symbol of the highest level of the Self.

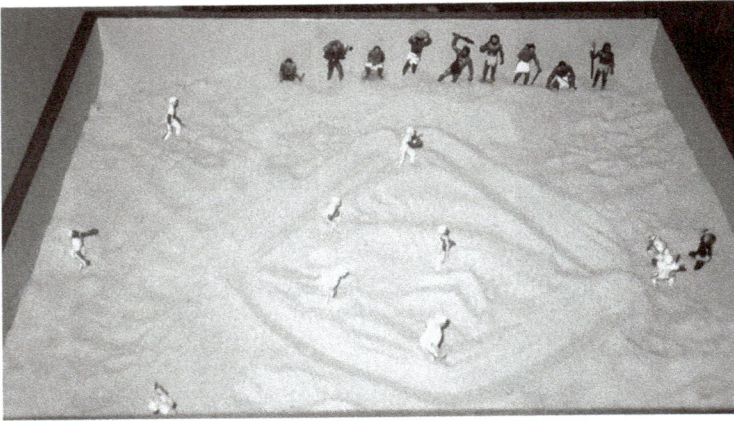

Figure 8.24 Tray of a 12-year-old boy

Figure 8.25

A 40-year-old Hispanic woman suffered four major losses in her life: her father died when she was nine, her grandmother when she was thirteen, and two brothers in a gang shoot-out when she was fifteen. She had spent much of her childhood and adolescence grieving these deaths. Now, on the anniversary of her father's death, she asked to make a sandplay.

Four shells serve as gravestone markers. A sundial shell and a tiny turtle are now able to be contained in one place. A nearby bicycle is available to take her on her way. The sundial shell suggests that time has passed and perhaps brings some closure to her mourning.

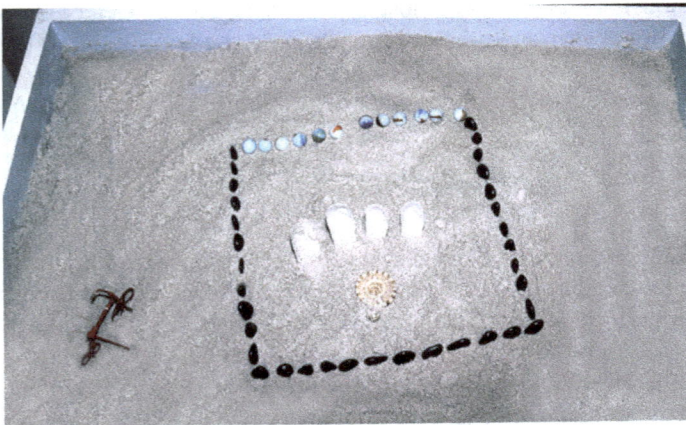

Figure 8.25 Tray of a 40-year-old woman

Figures 8.26 and 8.27

A highly skilled, hard-driving, 45-year-old businessman created this tray while playing like a child who is reluctant to use space. When he made this tray, he played in the sand for a long time, much like a two- or three-year-old, touching the sand and running it through his fingers. Then he chose one miniature – a death figure – and placed it on the right edge of the tray. In his first session, he had said that he had a life-long fear of dying suddenly of a heart attack, just as his father had. This man was two years old when he lost his father.

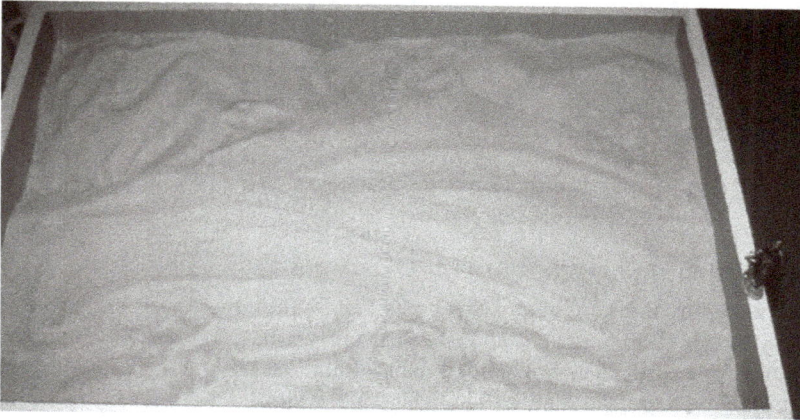

Figure 8.26 Tray of a 45-year-old man

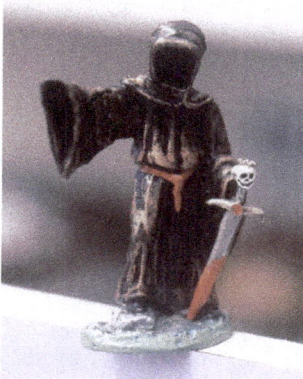

Figure 8.27 Tray of a 45-year-old man, detail

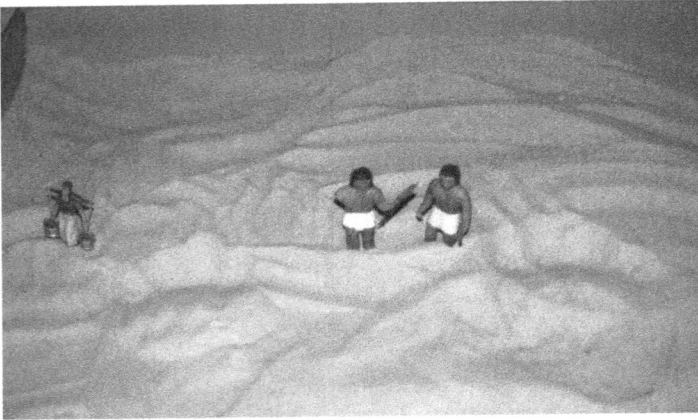

Figure 8.28 Tray of a 45-year-old man, six months later

Figures 8.28 and 8.29

This tray was created by the same man six months later. While the tray is still quite sparse – like that of a younger child – he does choose some fairly robust figures, which enliven the scene even though one of them is a wounded man without an arm. The milkmaid bringing milk might possibly be therapeutic milk to help heal his wounds.

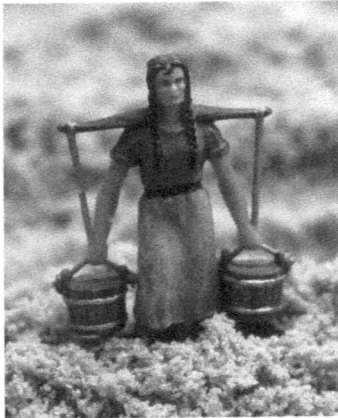

Figure 8.29 Tray of a 45-year-old man, six months later, detail

Gender influence on sandplay scenes

Several studies have found interesting gender differences in sandplay scenes. One is a classic study by Eric Erickson (1951); a second one is a study by Linn Jones (1986). Erickson's and

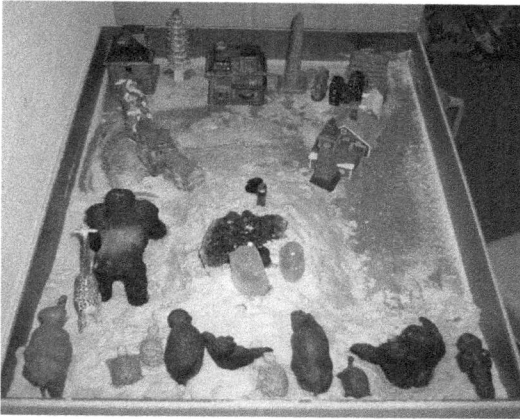

Figure 8.30 Tray of an eight-year-old boy

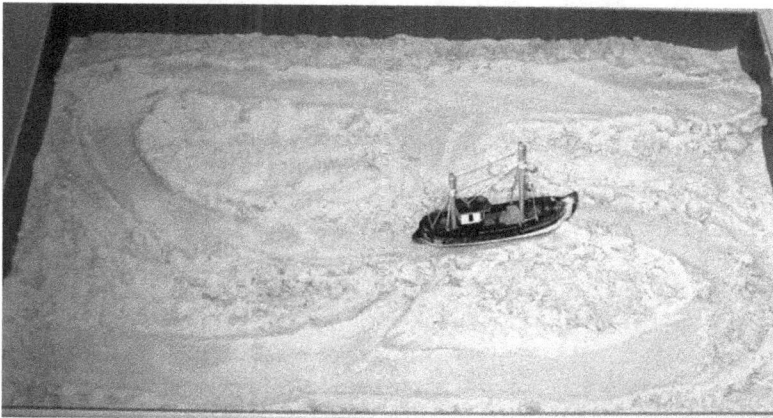

Figure 8.31 Tray of a six-year-old boy

Jones' research emphasized different aspects; however, they both agree that: (a) males tend toward aggressive scenes, and (b) females tend toward intimate, cooperative scenes.

Erickson found that boys' constructions use more blocks and vehicles at all ages. The blocks are used to erect structures, such as buildings and towers, and to build streets. Boys' stories often revolve around the dangers of collapse. **Figure 8.30** is one example from an eight-year-old boy. Boys' scenes also tend to involve more physical movement, and boys prefer miniatures that move or represent motion. **Figure 8.31** by a six-year-old boy is an example, with a boat and tracks made in the sand.

Girls employ blocks less frequently than boys, using them primarily to enclose a structure and to mark rooms in a house. Girls are more likely to use furniture and family figures in greater numbers than boys, e.g., **Figure 8.32**, created by an eight-year-old girl. Girls' scenes also tend to emphasize relationships among people, mainly family members. Fewer traumas

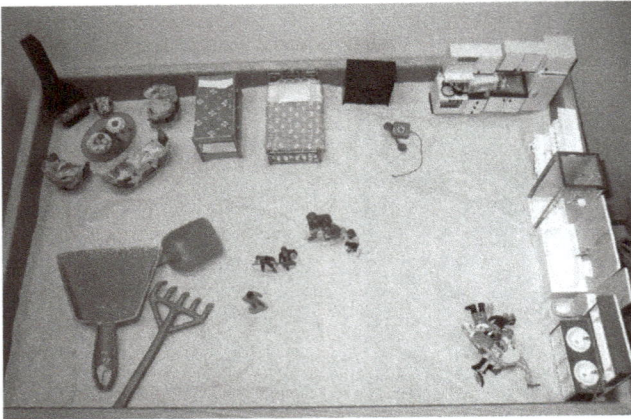

Figure 8.32 Tray of an eight-year-old girl

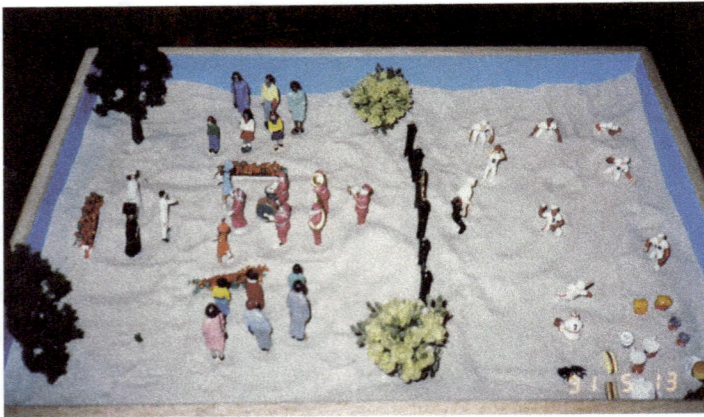

Figure 8.33 Tray of a ten-year-old girl

occur in the scenes. **Figure 8.33,** created by a ten-year-old girl, includes a fence. On one side a baseball game is taking place with lots of appropriate food for people watching the game. On the other side is a graduation scene with involvement by families.

Jones found that the structuring of sand worlds is similar for girls and boys, with two important exceptions. First, fewer boys manipulated the sand, i.e., boys tended to use the sand as a base, rather than moving the sand, especially between the ages of 7 and 13. Jones proposed that this finding suggested that the process of separation from the mother is more difficult for boys than for girls – an idea that resonates with Kalff's belief (1980) that work with the sand is related to "Mother Earth," the realm of instinct, nature, and the feminine.

Jones' second important finding was that there is a significant difference between boys and girls in how miniatures are used to display relationships in their dramatic play. Boys tend to engage in confrontive play and to represent that confrontation with a dynamic style (especially between two and seven years of age), while girls tend to focus on didactic relationships and family interactions, emphasizing cooperation (especially between five and seven years of age).

There were also indications that boys created fewer bodies of water than girls and also, in contrast to the girls, the boys created fewer islands. Jones' finding, that males tend toward aggressive play and that females tend toward more intimate, cooperative play, is consistent with Erikson's findings.

Little research has been conducted on the differences and similarities between the trays of adult men and women; however, Denkers (1985) found that more women than men have figures that relate to water.

Summary

Here, in outline form, are the major findings about age and gender influences on sandplay creations, discussed in this chapter.

Why is knowledge about sandplay developmental norms important?

- Helps therapists know what is typical and what is uncharacteristic for the client's age, and helps therapists to determine, for example, if the child is more or less advanced than other children at the same age
- If a child deviates from the norm, this may suggest a problem
- Sandplay pictures of disturbed adults and children exhibit patterns similar to those of young children

With increasing age (up to 12 years)

- A larger area of the tray is used
- A firmer sense of boundaries is evidenced by staying within the edges of the tray
- Control and coherence are enhanced
- Organization of miniatures within the tray becomes more structurally complex
- Contents of the tray become more realistic; miniatures are more integrated into the scene; and a time perspective is often included
- Individual differences in the content of the tray become more obvious. Under eight years old, trays are quite similar. After age eight, individual differences in the trays begin to emerge

Children aged two and three

- Demonstrate little or no control or focus; trays are usually chaotic, undifferentiated, and disorganized with no evidence of a cohesive perspective
- Typically they use only a small portion of the tray, paying no attention to the rest of the tray
- Ignore the tray's boundaries; figures are heaped and scattered across the room as well as within the tray
- Relationship between figures is "bizarre" and "highly subjective"
- Often poke, fling, or bury miniatures
- Sand is dropped and thrown inside and outside the tray

Children aged four and five

- Create trays that seem to be in transition:
- Some children use a small portion of the tray
- Others place toys at intervals throughout the tray
- Manage to have some coherent detail in separate areas within the tray
- Sand is used primarily for burying and un-burying figures
- Topics related to eating are common before the age of five; after five, farm scenes and many animals are used
- Use dramatic activity and move toys around in the tray, a "dynamic tray"
- Miniatures fight with each other
- Children sometimes make noises and speak for miniatures

Children aged six and seven

- By the age of six, children expand their ability to control (i.e., able to create the tray in the way they envision it, less chaotic)
- From six years old through eight, transport is a strong interest
- Starting at seven years, trees are used consistently
- "Normal" children begin to use the space out to all four sides of the tray
- The clinical population sometimes uses only a portion of the tray

Children aged ten and eleven

- Approaching ten years of age, control expands; one evidence of control is the use of fencing
- Ten years old is the peak age for using fences and other literal structures of control, such as signs

Children aged 12 through adulthood

- Starting at age 12, trays are similar to adult trays, which are usually complex with many miniatures
- Starting around age 12, fewer literal controls (i.e., fences) and more conceptual and symbolic controls are used (e.g., policemen). Also, topological features (e.g., mountains, streams) are used to control and unify a scene

General gender differences

Types of scenes:
- Females tend toward intimate, cooperative scenes
- Males tend toward aggressive, confrontational scenes

Displaying relationships:
- Girls tend to focus on both dyadic relationships and family interactions emphasizing cooperation (especially between five and seven years of age)
- Boys tend to engage in confrontational play and to represent that with a dynamic style (especially between two and seven years of age)

Gender differences characteristic of boys

- Boys' constructions use more blocks and vehicles at all ages
- The blocks are used to erect structures, such as buildings and towers and to build streets
- Boys' stories often revolve around the dangers of collapse
- Boys' scenes also tend to involve more physical movement
- Boys prefer miniatures that move or represent motion
- A common activity is moving cars and animals around streets, usually under the control of a toy policeman
- Fewer boys manipulate the sand, i.e., boys tend to use the sand as a base, rather than moving the sand (especially between seven and 13)
- Boys create fewer bodies of water than girls
- Boys tend to create few islands, contrary to girls

Gender differences characteristic of girls

- Girls employ blocks less frequently than boys, using them primarily to enclose a structure and to mark rooms in a house
- Girls are more likely to use furniture and family figures in greater numbers than boys
- Girls also tend to emphasize relationships among people, mainly family members
- Fewer traumas occur in scenes created by girls

Final comments

Looking at trays through the lens of age and gender can help identify which features are related to age, which to gender, and which to the uniqueness of the individual psyche – as well as to determine what is age appropriate, and what is not and may be a problem. Often the trays of adults who have experienced early trauma look surprisingly similar to those of young children. Being aware of developmental norms can be helpful in identifying adults who may have experienced a traumatic event at an early age, sometimes even giving an indication of the approximate age at which this event occurred.

Our intuitive view that sandplay can identify traumatic events is supported by Bowyer (1958) and by a study by Erik Erikson (1938). Erikson was interested in examining character development. He asked Harvard students to create dramatic scenes using miniatures. One of the most striking findings to come out of that study was that, even though the students were all English majors, they did not build scenes representing themes from literature or theater. Instead, very personal and intimate scenes emerged that could only be connected to traumatic events these students had experienced in their own childhoods. Their play with miniatures touched on early traumatic experiences, overshadowing these students' present issues.

We all realize that words are limited vehicles that do not allow the fullest and deepest expression of meaning. Words are the language of consciousness, but the unconscious speaks primarily in images. As a nonverbal technique, sandplay can bridge the cross-cultural communications of the soul. Like dreams, the images that emerge in the sand are, in essence, snapshots of the unconscious for us to behold and thus reach a deeper, more profound understanding.

Sandplay offers a unique opportunity to observe the unfolding development of the individual psyche. Sandplay is indeed one of those powerful facilitators that reaches into the deepest levels of the unconscious to access healing energies. Jung (in interview by Evans, 1977) succinctly addressed our personal responsibility in the healing of this alienated world when he said: "The world hangs by a thin thread and that thread is the human psyche." We believe that only through deep connection to our own psyches and struggling to heal ourselves can we strengthen that thin thread and become part of the healing fabric of this fragmented world.

References

Bowyer, L.R. (1956). A normative study of sand tray worlds. *Bulletin of British Psychological Society*. Summarized (1970) in L.R. Boyer, The Lowenfeld World Technique. Pergamon Press.

Bowyer, L.R. (1958). The sand tray world as a projective technique with mental defectives. *Journal of the Midland Mental Deficiency Society*, 4, 44–55.

Denkers, G.C. (1985). *An investigation of the diagnostic potential of sandplay utilizing Linn Jones' Developmental Scoring System*. Unpublished doctoral dissertation, Psychological Studies Institute, Pacific Grove Graduate School of Professional Psychology.

Erikson, E.H. (1938). Dramatic productions test. In H.A. Murray (Ed.), *Explorations in personality* (pp. 552–582). Oxford University Press.

Erikson, E.H. (1951). Sex differences in the play configurations of pre-adolescents. *American Journal of Orthopsychiatry*, 21, 667–692.

Evans, R.I. (1977). Interview with C. G. Jung: August 1957. In W. McGuire & R.F.C. Hull (Eds.), *Jung speaking: Interviews and encounters*. Princeton University Press.

Jones, L.E. (1986). *The development of structure in the world of expression: A cognitive-developmental analysis of children's "sand worlds."* (Doctoral dissertation, Pacific Graduate School of Psychology) Dissertation Abstracts International (University Microfilms No. 83-03178).

Jung, C.G. (1969). *The collected works of C.G. Jung: Structure & dynamics of the psyche* (Vol. 8, p. 190). Princeton University Press. (Originally published in 1927).

Kalff, D. (1980). *Sandplay: A psychotherapeutic approach to the psyche* (W. Ackerman, Trans.). Sigo Press.

Kamp, L.N.J., Ambrosius, A.M., & Zwaan, E.J. (1986). The World Test: Pathological traits in the arrangement of miniature toys. *Acta Psychiatrica Belgica*, 86(3), 208–219.

Kamp, L.N.J., & Kessler, E.G. (1970). The World Test: Developmental aspects of a play technique. *Journal of Child Psychology and Psychiatry*, 11, 81–108.

Chapter 9

Transference and countertransference in sandplay

Transference was first used by Freud "to describe what was happening when his women patients fell in love with him. He realized that his patients were repeating impulses and feelings in their relationship with him that they had experienced earlier, usually with parental figures" (Bradway & McCoard, 1997, p.31).

Jung believed that the client and therapist were involved in a two-way interaction in which both are impacted. It is the therapist's development as a person, rather than his/her theoretical knowledge, that is ultimately decisive in the treatment (Samuels, 1986). Jung also believed that, in the transference, the therapist stands in relation to the client both as a person and perhaps as a projection of the client's internal complex.

Historically, countertransference was viewed as a hindrance to therapeutic progress. However, the current view is that countertransference can also be helpful in the therapeutic endeavor. Countertransference is defined here as all the responses a therapist has to his/her client, including all feelings, fantasies, and interactions. Some of these reactions are conscious, while others are unconscious.

Transference and countertransference each can be positive or negative. Cunningham (2011) affirms that it is generally accepted in sandplay "that the countertransference container must be one of unconditional positive regard and warmth" (p.107). She cites Schore (2003) for additional emphasis, "positive transference and emotional safety are necessary to actually transform entrenched emotional-relational patterns in the brain." However, Cunningham reminds us that negative countertransference also can arise – what was called "a feeling against" by Bradway (1991) and Bradway & McCoard (1997). She advocates "emphasis on our own deep sensitivity in attending to the whole of our own – and our clients' – subjective experience" (p.106, also citing Wallin, 2007).

Historical views on transference and countertransference

Transference is a concept connected with psychoanalysis. Sigmund Freud observed and described this in the late 19th century. "He initially considered this phenomenon to be a hindrance to treatment, but his ideas evolved and he eventually came to recognize transference to be *an inherent necessity*," in psychoanalytic treatment (Suszek, Wegner & Maliszewski, 2015).

However, the issue of transference in child therapy has historically been controversial. Anna Freud believed that, since the child was in the process of developing a mother-child relationship, transference (i.e., transferring of client's feelings and behavior that have been generated by early experiences with significant others onto the therapist) was not a central issue in the therapeutic process with young children. On the other hand, Melanie Klein

(1952) believed that the analysis of transference was critical in understanding infantile traumas and deprivations because the child was currently in the grip of the living experience of the mother-child interaction.

Margaret Lowenfeld (1939) had yet another view on transference. She observed the client's central transference to be to the sand tray and materials themselves. Lowenfeld saw her role as one of understanding her clients' sand trays.

Kalff did not refer to transference in the classical sense of transferring old feelings onto the therapist; rather she was influenced by both Jung and Lowenfeld. For Kalff, "transference was the providing of space for the realization of one's potential" (Bradway, 1991, p.25). Kalff believed that, if a therapist could create a "free and protected space," this would facilitate a positive transference to the therapist that might, in turn, enhance the constellation of the Self. Over time, Kalff's views on transference evolved to include the idea that the relationship between client and therapist was sometimes directly expressed in the sand tray. Kalff began to see how sandplay creations themselves often directly referred to the client-therapist relationship. She saw, for example, how even a miniature chosen by a client might be depicting feelings that the client had toward the therapist.

Hayao Kawai (1985), a Japanese analyst, speaks of the connection between the sandplay therapist and client in terms of transference that occurs on the *Hara* level. In other words, a direct, nonverbal communication passes from the center (*Hara*) of one person to the center of the other person. More recently, Bradway and McCoard (1997), American analysts, use the term *co-transference* to designate the therapeutic feeling relationship between therapist and client. This feeling relationship is evoked by the sandplay experience as the sand picture is created. The transference takes place simultaneously, rather than sequentially as the term *transference-countertransference* suggests. Sometimes the sand picture produces an empowered form of relating as the therapist and the client view the sand picture together.

It is important to recognize and think about transference and countertransference in therapy; for example:

> The common occurrence of transference in life as well as in psychotherapy of the various orientations makes it inadvisable for therapists to ignore it. Transference is a vehicle of valuable information about the patient's functioning in relationships. This knowledge would very often be impossible to obtain from the patient in a different way because it is usually unconscious. (Suszek et al., 2015, p.374)

Increasingly, sandplay therapists have begun to look for and seriously take into account indications of transference in the trays. A client may even include a symbolic representation of the therapist in the sandplay picture. In this way, the state of the transference to the therapist has now become embodied.

It is important to give attention to the many ways sandplay pictures can speak to the therapeutic relationship. Our knowledge of how the transference makes itself known in sand creations has developed out of observing the variety of ways the transference becomes manifest in the sand.

Examples of transference and countertransference in sandplay

There are many ways that the transference relationship can be seen in a tray, including the way it is created. Some of the conscious indications of a transference relationship include:

- Client portrays the therapist in the sand
- Client identifies a particular object as the therapist
- Client creates a scene that he/she thinks will please (or displease) the therapist
- Sandplay miniatures are either openly shared or hidden from the therapist's view
- Client states that the content of the tray relates directly to the therapist

Some unconscious indications of the transference relationship are:

- Two similar miniatures often seem to portray feelings about the transference relationship
- Client creates a tray in which the content symbolically represents the relationship
- Placement or orientation of significant figures corresponds to where the therapist is sitting or standing
- Miniatures are treated in unusual ways, e.g., they are destroyed, stolen, envied, or valued
- The therapist's sandplay equipment (including the miniature collection, the display of the miniatures, or the quality of the sand) is criticized, praised, or compared to that of another therapist

The following trays are examples of some of the ways clients show their transference relationship to the therapist, together with some examples of countertransference:

Figure 9.1

This client consciously portrayed the therapist by sculpting the therapist's face in the sand.

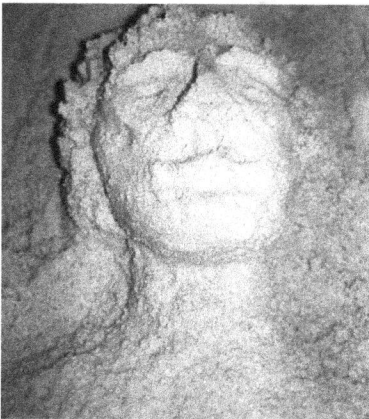

Figure 9.1 Example of transference

Figure 9.2

Another client consciously identified a miniature of Glinda, the good witch from *The Wizard of Oz*, as the therapist. He said, as he placed the miniature on the side of the tray and pointed at the therapist, "This is you – overseeing my land!" The therapist had strong countertransference reactions – flattered to be the good witch but not wanting that power.

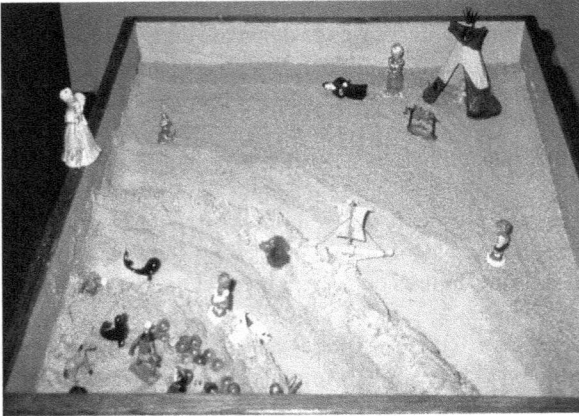

Figure 9.2 Example of transference

Figure 9.3

This client created a sand picture that she thought would please the therapist.

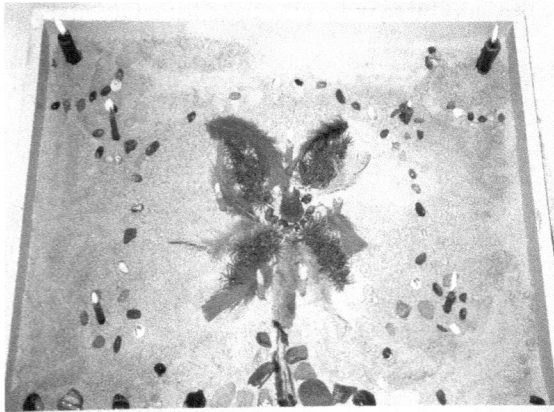

Figure 9.3 Example of transference

Figure 9.4

Some clients create trays to displease or shock their therapist. This client first resisted sand-play, then decided to make a tray. She had been in therapy for a year or more before she even approached sandplay, although she often talked about wanting and not wanting to create a sand-play. When she decided it was now time to create a sandplay, she stood at the tray for a long time and then slowly picked these three objects. She placed a queen near the center of the tray, a soldier with raised sword behind the queen, and a wolf in front of the queen. She then moved the wolf to bite the queen. After she finished the sandplay, she stood and looked at it for a long time.

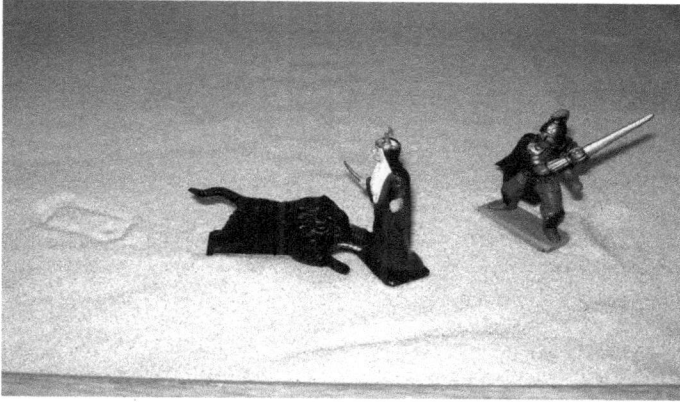

Figure 9.4 Example of transference

In reflecting on my countertransference feeling, I wondered: "Did I push her too much to create a tray?" Earlier in therapy, she described being abused badly by her mother. Was creating a sandplay too exposing, too threatening, for her? I chose not to ask her because I felt a question might be an intrusion on my part. She did continue in therapy, and she felt it was helpful to her; however, this was the only tray she created during her treatment.

Figures 9.5 and 9.6

Sometimes a client makes a special point of openly showing a miniature or hiding it from the therapist; this behavior often relates to the transference. While creating this tray, the 37-year-old Latina woman asked me to leave the room. She said she would call me when she had finished hiding something. When I returned, she told me that I could only see what she had hidden after she left the office.

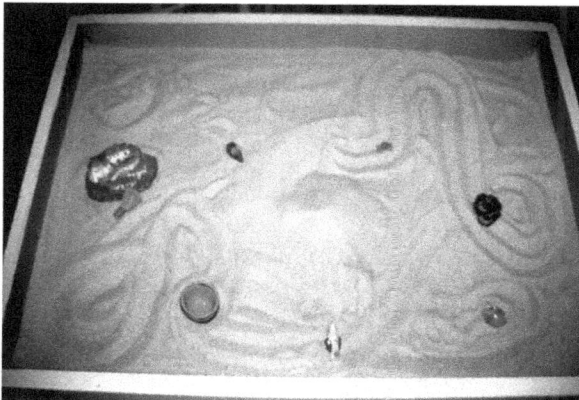

Figure 9.5 Tray of a 37-year-old woman

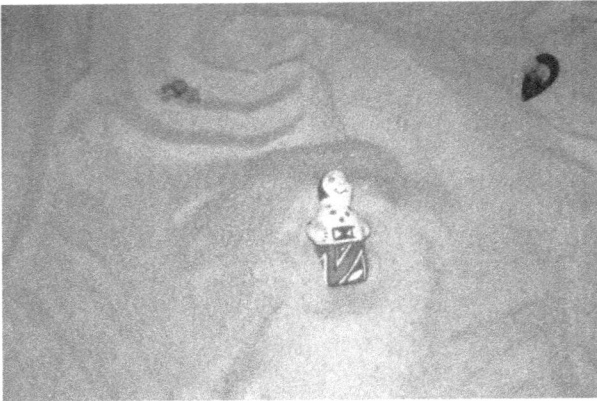

Figure 9.6 Tray of a 37-year-old woman, detail

This tray seems almost a complete opposite to the previous example and yet similar. On the positive side, it clearly differentiates the two of us. On the not so positive side, there is a defense against merging – and rejection of me as her companion on the journey. When she asked me to go to the other room, I felt pushed aside, rejected from being part of her experience. I also realized that her request was an important individuation statement. When I later unburied this figure, it was clear to me that she had left a wise woman from her own culture and that she wanted me to hold it and think of her.

Figure 9.7

The content of the tray in Figure 9.7 relates directly to the therapist. This client selected a plant for his sand picture that was located in the waiting room, outside of the sandplay room. The plant was a personal item belonging to me. My countertransference was both negative and positive. When he left the therapy room and went into the waiting room, I wondered to

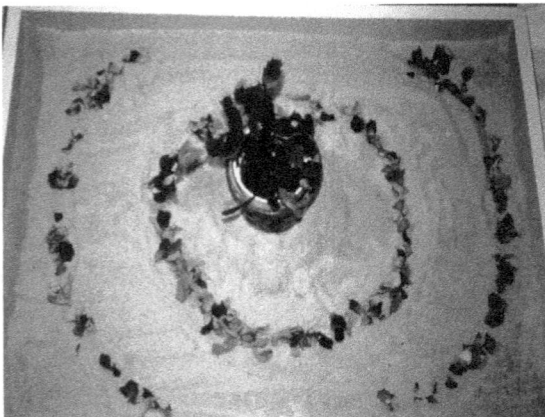

Figure 9.7 Tray that led to countertransference

myself, "What in the world is he going to do?" I was surprised at my feelings. I wondered, "Why is he transgressing the boundaries of our sandplay experience? Why does he need even more miniatures than I already have in this room?" It was helpful to realize that this was a transference and countertransference situation. That insight helped me deepen my understanding. He needed even more of me than what I was giving him in that room.

Figures 9.8 and 9.9

A transference relationship is also often symbolized by the placement of two matching miniatures in the tray. Such a placement portrays the client's feelings toward and identification with the therapist. This tray was created by a 45-year-old woman, near the end of therapy. In

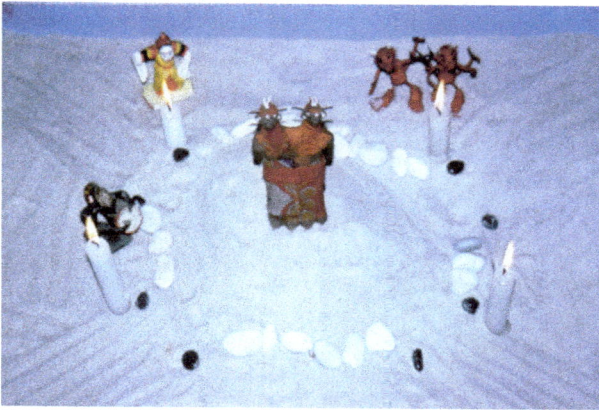

Figure 9.8 Tray of a 45-year-old woman

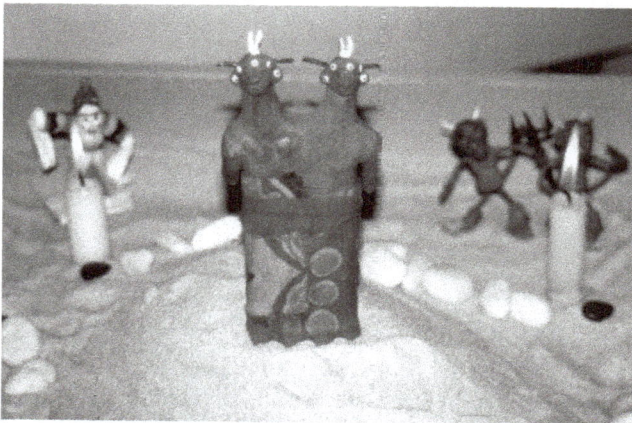

Figure 9.9 Tray of a 45-year-old woman, detail

the previous month she gave me this conjoint twin figure as a gift. Now she placed it at the center of the tray, suggesting a union and close identification with me. Because she was ending therapy, I discussed this with her. She told me that she would always hold me in her heart. To myself, I wondered if this was bad or good. I think this was her way of complimenting me, but I also wanted her to feel strong without me. I decided I wasn't going to ask her to explore it at her last session. I thanked her and said I thought she was a very strong woman and that I admired her (which was true).

Figure 9.10

In the tray, a 12-year-old girl placed a wounded young female figure on a stretcher with a doctor and nurse nearby. On an unconscious level, the content of the tray symbolically represents the relationship with me. This girl is unconsciously stating that she is getting the treatment she needs. I could feel her relaxing as she made the tray. In her subsequent sessions after making this tray, I felt a new sense of trust on her part, and I felt closer and more relaxed with her as well.

This also represents a "please the therapist tray." The client was very anxious to have a positive reaction from me. I had mixed feelings about how to respond. Normally I make neutral, observational comments and sometimes ask a few questions about a tray. I don't usually make reinforcing or evaluative statements.

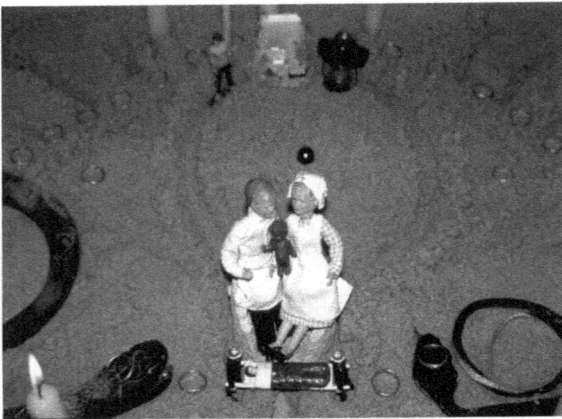

Figure 9.10 Tray of a 12-year-old girl

Figure 9.11

This is an example of an "unconscious message tray," with a negative transference, which was created unintentionally. One semester, while teaching a graduate class in child counseling, I decided to give the class an opportunity to observe a child making a sand tray. I asked David and his mother for their permission for him to create a sand tray in this teaching situation. This is the tray he made. There are three enclosures, one with pigs, one with sheep,

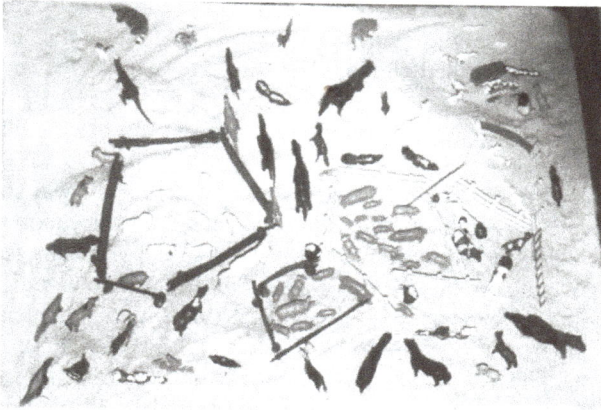

Figure 9.11   David's first tray

and one with pigs and cattle. I noted that the number of pigs in the first pen was exactly the number of students that were present in the class that evening. I believe this was his way of containing the situation.

Figure 9.12

Two days later, at David's next therapy session, when he created this tray, I realized how upsetting the previous teaching situation had been for him. He told me then that he had experienced his tray-creating experience in front of an audience as an intrusion into his sacred space.

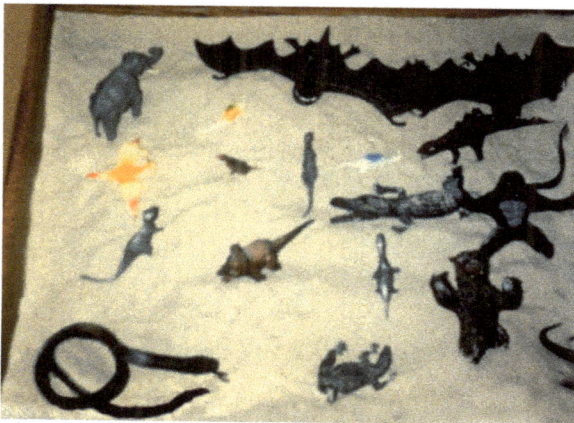

Figure 9.12   David's subsequent tray

This boy's family often fought among themselves. In this tray, he placed three bats (which he named Mommy, Dad, and Baby) and said that all of the animals were fighting. As he had them fighting, he said, "the baby bat thought the terrible snake was nice, but it hurt him; it killed him. Then the parents got mad and killed all the other animals. Then they found that the baby bat was still alive."

At this point, David carefully separated all the animals and commented that he liked it better when everybody was happy.

I think it was significant that David placed the large snake closest to where I was sitting. Both the placement of the snake and his comment that the terrible snake was nice, but it hurt him communicated to me: "I thought you were nice and I trusted you, but you betrayed me and it makes me mad." I was relieved to see that his own protective defenses emerged at this moment of anger, and he was able to separate and remove the various frightening elements without destroying the entire experience.

After his session, I thought a great deal about his tray, and I decided I would ask him about this at our next session. After he settled in at the next session, I asked, "I wonder if you felt angry about having to make a sandplay for the class?" He nodded yes.

I believe that my understanding of his anger at me and my acceptance helped move the therapy to an even deeper level, but I made the decision to never make the same mistake again. After this event, David had a number of therapy sessions. Near the end of therapy, his parents reported to me that he doing well in school and had made some good friends. However, I couldn't forget the mistake I made by asking him to expose his feelings and unconscious thoughts to others.

References

Bradway, K. (1991). Transference and countertransference in sandplay therapy. *Journal of Sandplay Therapy*, *1*(1), 25–43.

Bradway, K., & McCoard, B. (1997). *Sandplay: Silent workshop of the psyche*. Routledge.

Cunningham, L. (2011). Countertransference in sandplay: The heart and the mind of a loving, attuned other. *Journal of Sandplay Therapy*, *20*(1), 105–115.

Kawai, H. (1985). Introduction: On transference in sandplay therapy. In H. Kawai & Y. Yamanaka (Eds.), *Studies of Sandplay Therapy in Japan* (Vol. II, pp. iii–xi). Seishin-Shoboh.

Klein, M. (1952). The origin of transference. *International Journal of Psycho-Analysis*, *33*, 433–438.

Lowenfeld, M. (1939). The World pictures of children: A method of recording and studying them. *British Journal of Medial Psychology*, *18*(1), 65–101.

Samuels, A. (1986). *A critical dictionary of Jungian analysis*. Routledge & Kegan Paul.

Schore, A. (2003). *Affect regulation and the repair of the self*. W.W. Norton & Company.

Suszek, H., Wegner, E., & Maliszewski, N. (2015). Transference and its usefulness in psychotherapy in light of empirical evidence. *Roczniki Psychologiczne (Annals of Psychology)*, *18*(3), 363–380. http://czasopisma.tnkul.pl/index.php/rpsych/article/view/673

Wallin, D.J. (2007). *Attachment in psychotherapy*. The Guilford Press.

Chapter 10

Sandplay and alchemy

This chapter includes a very unique case that dramatically depicts the living connection between the alchemical process and sandplay. The unfolding sandplay process of a six-year-old boy (named "Peter" for this narrative) displayed many similarities to the ancient, archetypical alchemical process. In retrospect, Peter's journey was a necessary one. Only through an alchemical process was he able to access the deepest layers of the unconscious and thus transform the negative emotions buried there.

C.G. Jung wrote extensively about the similarity between alchemy and the psychotherapeutic process. Alchemy, analytical psychology, and sandplay have much in common; they all attempt to forge a link between the conscious mind and the world of the unconscious. Also, both alchemy and sandplay involve the manipulation of concrete materials through unique processes in order to coagulate, or bring together and realize, the images of the unconscious.

Alchemy was an early form of science, a proto-science, whose goal was to transform base metals into gold. However, it was far more than that. Alchemists thought of themselves as committed to a sacred work – a search for supreme and ultimate value – as symbolized by the gold. In reaching this goal, the character of the alchemist played a central role. Not only was the knowledge of this ancient discipline important, but the alchemist had to possess certain personal characteristics, such as patience, perseverance, courage, and discipline. Often, unbeknown to them, as the alchemists labored in the search for the key to the transformation of physical matter, the process was also transforming their own souls.

According to Jung (1969, originally written in 1944), the purpose of alchemical work (which the alchemists called "the opus") was not only to make gold but also to rescue the human soul from a meaningless and chaotic existence. Jung believed that this ancient work deeply affected the alchemists' own psyches in profound ways. As they worked, immersed in various processes in the alchemical laboratory, they were working at the most profound level of the unconscious to reach psychic gold – that often-hidden part of ourselves that Jung calls the Self.

Sandplay, similar to its ancient predecessor, alchemy, gives shape to unconscious content and directly affects the dynamics of both conscious and unconscious processes. The pictures in sandplay are reflections of inner images that emerge into consciousness. However, what is constellated in the tray also affects the unconscious. Thus, a cyclical process unfolds. Dora Kalff (1980), the originator of sandplay, states that the healing experience is a direct consequence of relating to internal images and giving them concrete form. At times, sandplay sets into motion profound and mysterious happenings, as illustrated in the case of six-year-old Peter discussed in this chapter.

Jung's writings on alchemy have been amplified by several writers. One that has influenced this chapter is Edward Edinger. In his book, *The Anatomy of the Psyche*, Edinger (1985) identifies and discusses seven operations in the alchemical process – *solutio, calcinatio, sublimatio, coagulatio, separatio, mortificatio*, and *coniunctio. Coniunctio* is the final stage or the culmination of the opus – reaching the gold.

Even though Edinger points out that other writers have identified somewhat different alchemical operations and that not all of his seven identified operations have to be present in order for transformation to take place, in the sandplay case of Peter, all seven of these stages were present.

Some background about Peter: the initial meeting was with Peter's parents. They wanted him in therapy because of their concern about his habitual displays of defiance, anger, and hostility. They said that Peter was often rude and actively defied or refused to comply with adults' requests or rules. According to his parents, Peter had a "dark side." At times, he could be very mean, almost cruel, especially when someone was "on his turf." For example, if a visiting friend happened to be winning a game, Peter would fly into a rage. His parents said that Peter was a large child and could easily bully others into letting him win or, if they did not, he would stop playing and sulk in a corner. They also described him as easily frustrated. For example, when he was first trying to learn Nintendo, he would scream, cry, and shout his frustration. Finally, he would throw the controls and give up in anger. Then, after a few weeks, he would try again. He finally mastered the game after a substantial period of time, and now it seemed that he couldn't get enough of it. His mother had to monitor both Nintendo and television because on his own he would choose to do nothing else.

According to his parents, Peter had a difficult birth and was delivered by an unplanned caesarian section – after the birth process had begun. From the very beginning, he was difficult to soothe and had a high reactivity to any change in stimuli, particularly to noise and light.

Both of his parents were college graduates. Peter's father, a successful executive in the film business, was often away on location. His mother, a homemaker, often felt tired and "beat up." Although she tried not to get into a power struggle with Peter, there were still daily conflicts marked by his tears and rages. At times, though, she said that Peter could be quite kind. Peter has a baby sister who was born when he was five-and-a-half years old. He seems to love her, and he enjoys watching and playing with her. Around the time of the birth of his sister, the family moved to a new home.

In school, Peter functioned very well. His achievements in reading and arithmetic were outstanding, and his behavior in the classroom was usually appropriate for his age. However, at school play time, he went between extremes of making trouble and isolating himself. For example, he had recently become very angry when he was "tagged" in dodge ball. He refused to leave the center of the circle and shouted loudly at the girl who had tagged him, yelling that she had cheated. Eventually, a teacher intervened, and Peter ran to the far side of the playground to kick stones against the fence.

After hearing his parents' concerns, I observed Peter at school. However, that day his behavior was quite ordinary. His teacher told me about his temper tantrums and difficulty in making friends. She also said that Peter was probably an academically gifted child.

Based on the reports of his parents and teacher and observations in therapy, Peter clearly met the criteria for an ICD-10 diagnosis on Axis I: Oppositional Defiant Disorder.

In addition to involving Peter in sandplay therapy, additional therapy techniques included: play therapy, behavioral therapy, relaxation and self-talk training, visualization, bibliotherapy, and art. He was in weekly therapy sessions for almost two-and-a-half years.

Early in therapy, Peter's sandplay pictures suggested that he was trying to work through dark, difficult, and unresolved issues that raged within him. Eventually, it was his work in the sand that both activated and ultimately was the vehicle he needed to transform his dark, instinctual elements, so that he could better function in the world. With the use of these new connections, the ego was able to relate to the Self, which helped him develop in a more harmonious way. As his therapy progressed, it became clear that Peter was trying to work through the dark, difficult, and unresolved issues that raged within him.

The following are 14 of the 25 scenes Peter created during his sandplay process (numbered 1–14 here). His first three trays are very typical for boys in therapy. The fourth tray is quite different. Then, starting with the fifth tray, the beginning of the seven operations in the alchemical process is displayed in his work. However, it is not until his final tray that all seven operations join together to create transformation at the deepest level of the psyche.

Figure 10.1 (Tray 1, July 14)

A chaotic situation is evident in this sandplay. A war is in progress, reminiscent of Kalff's *Fighting* stage. There is fragmentation, but here, amid the war, is a newsstand! What is the news? Perhaps it had something to do with his beginning therapy. It is interesting that he placed the newsstand in the upper right corner; sometimes this corner is associated with new development.

This tray represents several layers of Peter's development – as well as the possibility of new development. Snakes represent the primal level, while the collective level is represented by the knights, civil war soldiers, and king's guards. According to Peter, the castle is under siege and the two tanks and cannons, pointing at each other, are on opposite sides, suggesting chaotic and conflicted feelings. Peter then placed a golden crown on the head of a soldier. However, only later in therapy did it become apparent that the element of gold would be very important in his search for a stable self.

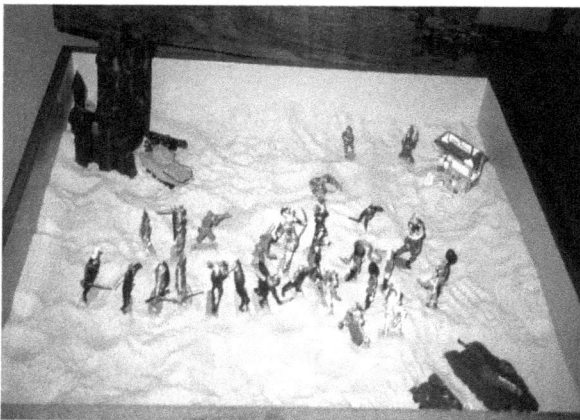

Figure 10.1 Tray 1

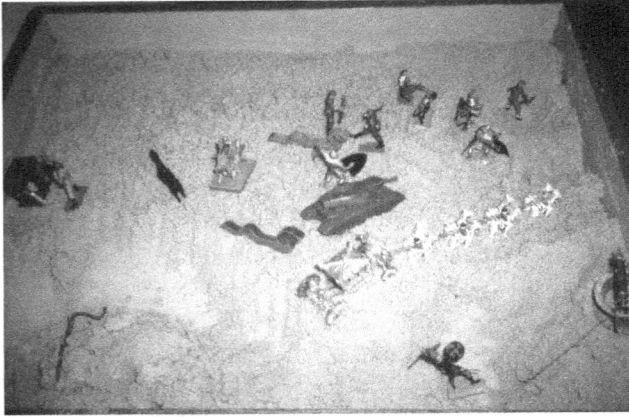

Figure 10.2 Tray 2

Figure 10.2 (Tray 2, July 14)

Peter created both this and Tray 1 in his second session. This tray included images of gold and finding a path, and the tray begins to show some movement, as expressed in his use of a golden horse-drawn carriage. Also, the use of the water wheel in the well indicates that Peter is attempting to reach inward to access and activate the energies of the unconscious.

Over the next few weeks, Peter created several more sand scenes. All of them depicted chaos and struggle, which is quite typical of six-year-old boys.

Figure 10.3 (Tray 3, November 15)

This tray, created about four months after his first two trays, is full of struggle, but there are beginning attempts to bridge the frightening elements of the unconscious. Peter was a child

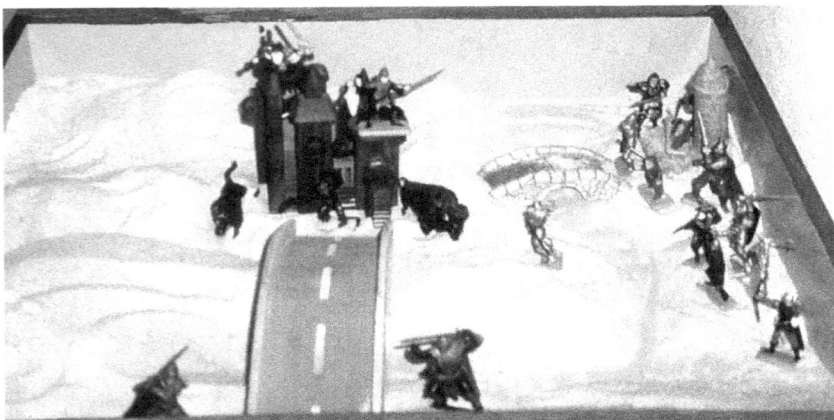

Figure 10.3 Tray 3

who often demonstrated his anger with uncontrollable rage. This picture reveals some of what is underneath the rage – primitive, destructive elements that he has no control over – the large, powerful aggressive fighters. He calls them "bad guys." He is trying to bridge, control, and understand them. The two bridges and two buffalos suggest that instinctual elements are guarding the more primitive parts of him. In Native American lore, the buffalo symbolizes supernatural power, strength, and fortitude. It was good to see that type of energy in this tray. Miniatures that are somewhat less threatening (than the bad guys up front) are off to the left side. The castle itself is full of aggressive elements containing both bad guys and good guys. It is not clear which side reigns. Up to this point, Peter's sandplay pictures are quite typical of boys in therapy. His trays suggest that this is a boy who is struggling to develop an ego and fight the younger, primitive aspects of himself.

Figure 10.4 (Tray 4, November 29)

Peter created a very different tray two weeks later. The intensity with which he put this network of pipes together was impressive. Clearly, he was undergoing important structural work in his psyche. His process seemed much deeper and suggested that perhaps a profound and mysterious process was being set in motion. The piping and cords were perhaps connected to his caesarian birth. Was this the beginnings of a reorganized ego? Later, looking back on this tray from an alchemical perspective, it appears that Peter was creating a new path through which his energy could flow in an interconnected way.

After this tray, Peter stopped creating trays for about four months. Instead, during the sessions, he spent much of his time crawling through the mazes he created, using two large plastic tunnels in the therapy office. As he placed barriers in and around the tunnels, which he had to struggle over and under to find his way through, I wondered if his behavior possibly paralleled the struggle he must have had at birth. His birth had not been a successful struggle; it had been necessary for others to help him before he could complete it. Here, in therapy, he at last had the chance to complete the birthing struggle over and over again, at his own pace. I knew he needed to do this with his own physical body. This work laid the foundation for a new process to begin – the alchemical process.

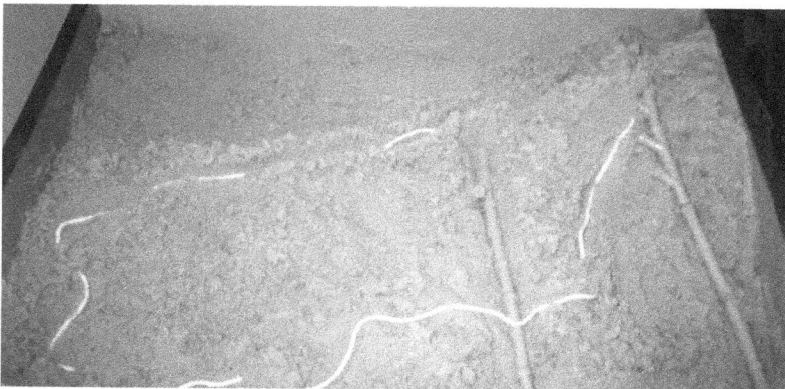

Figure 10.4 Tray 4

Figures 10.5 and 10.6 (Tray 5, April 11 of the following year)

After five months of almost weekly play therapy sessions, Peter took a big step forward in his next sandplay creation. He now was able to bridge two sand trays!

Using more energy than in previous sandplays, he moved large amounts of sand to create an unusual scene of water and shoreline. The moving of the sand suggests that this is a child with good mental capacity whose inner resources of imagination are becoming more available. Now, there is more space for him to work on his issues. This sandplay reflects the work and struggle that had been going on in his play therapy sessions, as well as in his previous sand pictures.

There are several alchemical operations represented in this tray, but the most relevant is the alchemical stage of *solutio* (additional stages will be discussed later in connection with Peter's other trays). *Solutio* pertains to water. Some alchemists believed that *solutio* was the

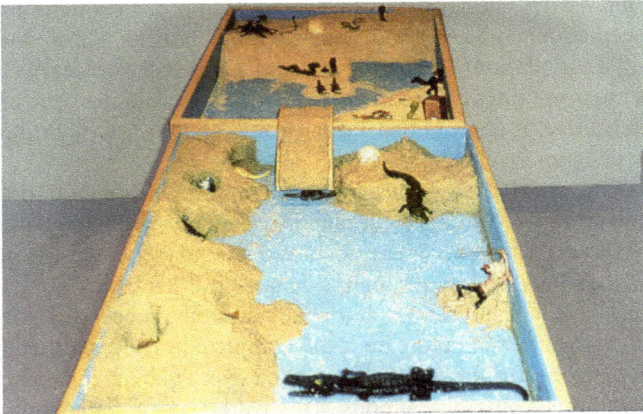

Figure 10.5 Tray 5

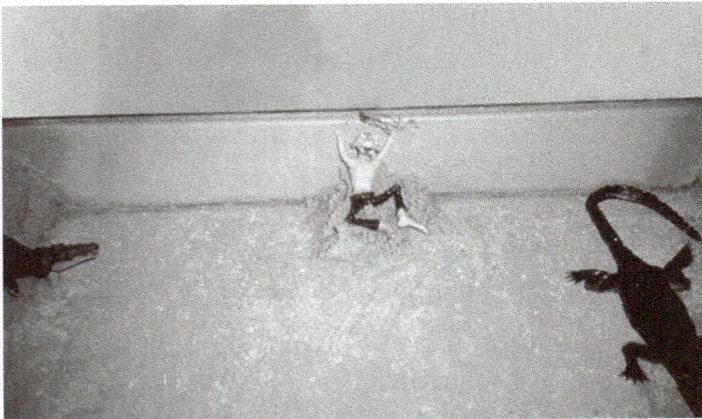

Figure 10.6 Tray 5 detail

root of alchemy. According to Edinger (1985), one ancient alchemist advised: "Until all be made water, perform no operation." *Solutio* often meant the return of differentiated matter to its original and undifferentiated state, *prima materia*, or (in English) its first or primal material."

Solutio has a twofold effect: it causes one form to disappear or regress to *prima materia*, and then a new, regenerated form emerges. In the human condition, the fixed, static aspects of the personality retard change. For transformation to proceed, these fixed aspects must often first be dissolved or reduced to the psyche's *prima materia* – that is, the painful feelings that produce the suffering – before new aspects can arise. As therapists know, clients often need to cry before change can take place.

This tray illustrates a time of tremendous reorganization. In talking about his tray, Peter said that a big hurricane had come and the man and animals were spread around the earth. He then proceeded to make several caves for some of the animals, creating a contained space for these energies to reside and find protection.

His selection of a man with agony on his face was striking. The man's agony may connect with Peter's own struggle and pain. The wet fury of the hurricane could represent archetypal energy – the energy that tormented him – reducing his anger and rage to *prima materia* while moving him along on his journey.

Symbols of death are present in this tray (the coffin and skulls), but there is also the possibility of movement and connection, as symbolized by the large bridge between the two trays, and the possibility of transformation, as symbolized by the snakes.

The two alligators are prominent in this tray. As Peter moved the smaller alligator toward the bigger one, he said, "The son and dad are going to fight each other." However, the actual encounter did not happen in the tray, and he moved the smaller alligator back to its original place.

Figure 10.7 (Tray 6, June 20)

Approximately two months later, Peter created this sandplay picture with a mandala-shaped mound, complete with cartoon characters, Wiley Coyote and the Roadrunner (the

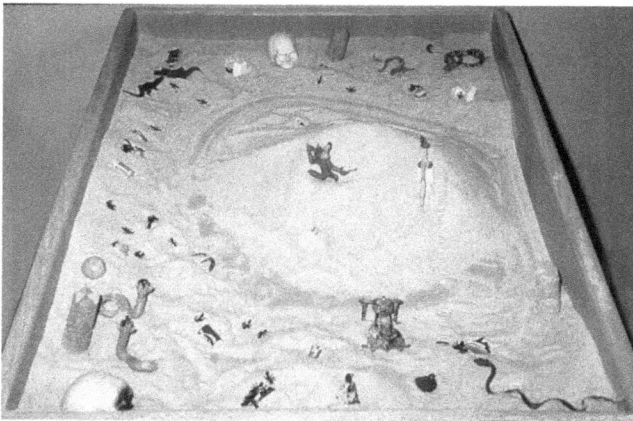

Figure 10.7 Tray 6

ultimate survivor). Peter now has the ability to form a circular arrangement in the sand, a new statement that he had never made before. Something new had been born within him. Perhaps he has now created a new relationship with his own psyche, a new ability to bring parts of his psyche together. Certainly the potential for a coming together (a joining) is visible in this tray.

Still, many fragmented parts are scattered around the mound; these need to be integrated as well. The primitive king and queen figures are standing amid material that was used in earlier trays. This tray raises the question, "will Peter be able to integrate so much fragmented, chaotic material and move these elements into a new order that was clearly emerging in the center of the tray?"

The chaotic material surrounding the mound is more *prima materia* that needs to be transformed. All these chaotic elements – more than any six-year-old should have to deal with – are now in the hands of a larger dynamic. His psyche was in an activated state of reorganizing itself. Through his sandplay process, he was searching to order and reconfigure his internal state.

Figure 10.8 (Tray 7, July 29)

Five weeks later, more had come together. This sandplay evoked a strong emotional experience in Peter. He demonstrated a great sense of accomplishment in building this central mountain structure and in filling the cup (in the background) with wet sand and placing it on top. This structure, and his emotion in creating it, represent a birthing of a new and solid ego. Now, his new internal structure can incorporate both light and dark aspects. The *Star Wars* miniatures (both the good guys and the bad guys) are in one central organized structure. Land bridges are present. It appears that he is now able to bridge both worlds; however, perhaps, more on one side than the other.

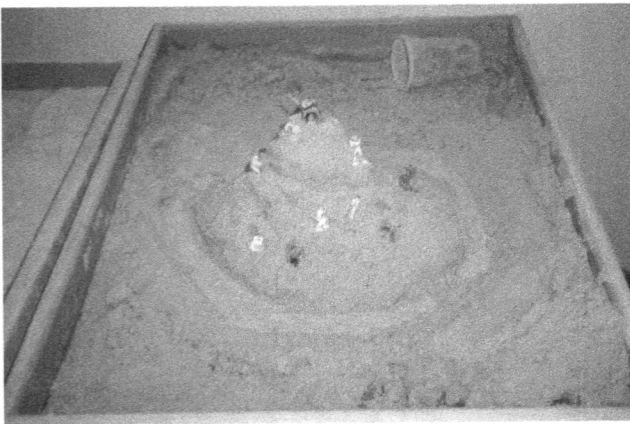

Figure 10.8 Tray 7

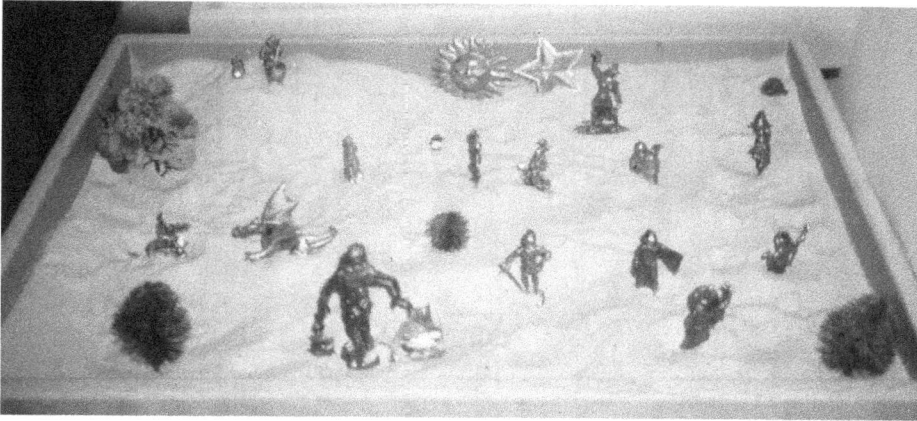

Figure 10.9 Tray 8

Figure 10.9 (Tray 8, August 5)

Peter created this tray the following week It is very different from any tray he had created before. Perhaps this tray was possible because of the previous tray.

Peter used greenery for the first time. The flowering tree, in the right back corner, is located in almost the same place as the newsstand in his first tray. This suggests that a deep, internal vegetative level of growth had been activated. Second, almost all of the figures are made of base metal. Metal was a core common element of the *prima materia* in alchemy; it was the original material from which gold was to be created. The most striking feature of metal is its heaviness and solidity; it is a good symbol of concrete, earthy reality. Two items in the tray, the sun and the star, have already attained the ultimate state of transformation into gold. A third figure is in the tray: a golden, primitive person mixing something in a cauldron.

This tray suggests that Peter was going through a deep process and working like an ancient alchemist in his inner laboratory. Despite the dark elements here, they are overseen by the light of the sun and the star. This and the previous tray indicate that the Self had become manifest and now, in this tray, the Self is working to transmute these base metals into gold.

Figure 10.10 (Tray 9, November 22)

This tray was created just after Peter's seventh birthday. He placed seven small candles, as well as a large one in the tray. (The seventh small candle is on the left side but outside the picture.) With the myriad of lighted candles, Peter now seems able to shed light upon his frustration and anger. Jung (1968, p.190) refers to a multitude of lights as "the seeds of light broadcast in the chaos."

Peter has clearly moved further into an alchemical process. In this tray, the second, third, and fourth alchemical stages appear: *calcinatio, sublimatio,* and *coagulatio.* The alchemical stage of *calcinatio* refers to an encounter with fire. Fire has a purging or purifying effect. It purges primitive feelings so the ego can connect to its own proper level of energy and functioning. Psychologically, *calcinatio* refers to the ordeal of enduring intense emotions. If the ego can hold together, the ordeal ultimately has consolidating effects.

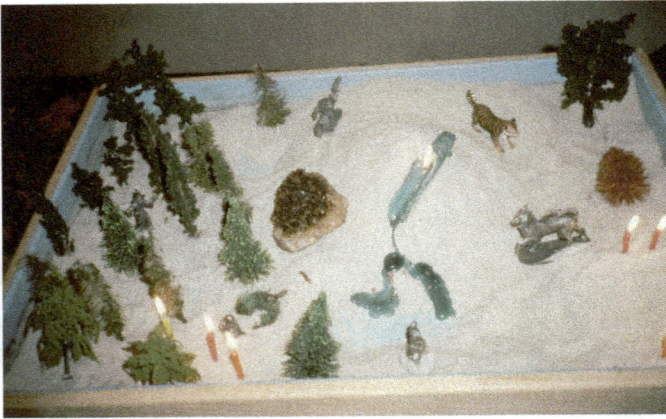

Figure 10.10 Tray 9

Fire can also heat up other substances and, when this happens, some substances evaporate into the air. In alchemy, this is called *sublimatio*. For example, water is heated, then turns into steam and evaporates into air. Other substances, when heated, melt and change form, sometimes clotting together. This is the alchemical stage of *coagulatio*, which refers to the coming together of a substance.

In this sandplay, both processes occur when fire heats the central blue candle, causing smoke to ascend into the air (*sublimatio*). Then fire melts the candle, and molten wax flows down the hill, blending and attaching itself to the earth (*coagulatio*). Edinger (1985) says that *coagulatio* is a "process that turns something into earth." Symbolically, *coagulatio* is the constellation of a cohesive self.

Figure 10.11 (November 29)

In this tray, one week later, further development of the stage of *coagulatio* occurs. Peter makes sure that two streams of molten blue candle wax join together and firmly coagulate at the bottom of the hill, pouring into the lake. As this connection is established, he uses humans for the first time (Before this, Peter used only cartoon and archetypal figures, e.g., knights). Now, as more of his ego is established, symbolized by the coming together of the blue molten wax, he is able to access and utilize a more ordinary grounded symbol: Native American people, who live in a natural, earthy way. In the past, the primitive aspect of his psyche had been expressed in more violent and aggressive ways, in trays depicting themes of fighting and death. Now, he is able to progress on his journey in a yellow canoe, as two mother figures are placed in clearly distant places separate from him (I wondered to myself if these two figures were perhaps his mother and me?). Here, too, are more images of fire and cooking, again suggesting the alchemical stage of *calcinatio*. Several snakes are in this tray, suggesting a powerful potential for transformation that I felt was so alive in him.

For three months, Peter did not create sandplay pictures. Instead he used our time together to talk about friends, family, and school successes and problems.

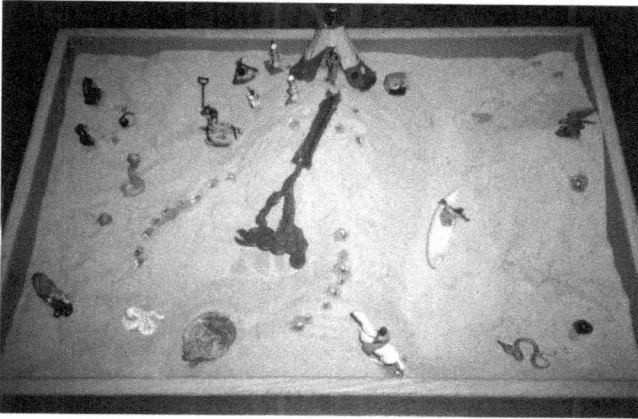

Figure 10.11 Tray 10

Figure 10.12 (February 27, following year)

Three months later, Peter again stood before the sand tray and then created a totally new form. This sculpted form might have evolved out of the previously amorphous coagulated wax in his past tray. Peter subjected the sand (his *prima materia*) to a series of operations and changes (i.e., *coagulatio* [becoming earth] and *calcinatio* [fire]) and created a completely new form – one he had not made before.

In this tray, the fifth alchemical stage of *separatio* (separation) occurs. In *separatio*, order is brought forth out of confusion. In a process that is similar to a theme in creation myths where the cosmos or the world is born out of chaos, Peter separated his sculpted figure from the rest of the sand and gave it its own separate form.

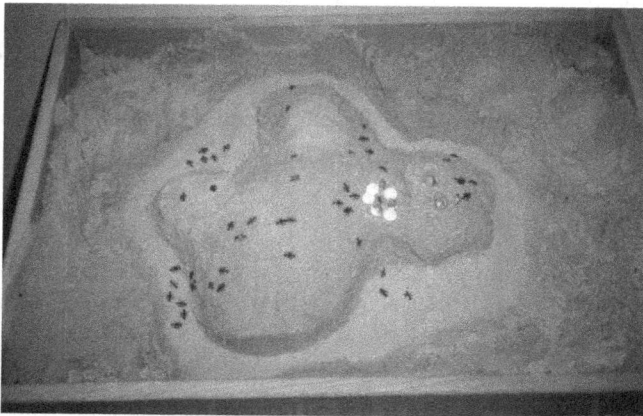

Figure 10.12 Tray 11

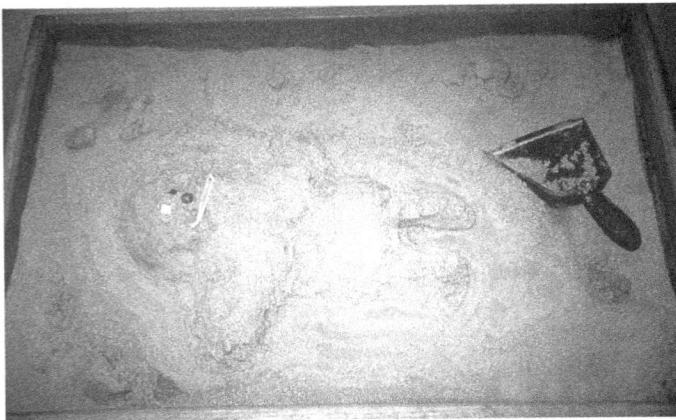

Figure 10.13 Tray 12

Peter's placement of ants on his figure was interesting. Ants are the most ordinary of insects. While ants operate on an instinctual level, they also participate in a fully developed collective community with clearly identified roles. One of their hallmarks and characteristics is the creation of elaborate tunnels in soil.

In therapy, Peter was also beginning to talk about himself and his life in more specific ways than ever before. During his sessions, he was also engrossed in artwork and play therapy. On the same day that he created this tray, he drew an elaborate labyrinth on paper, suggesting that much more was going on internally than could be seen from merely observing him. His own underpinnings were being created in more separate – and complex – ways. This work is similar to the internal work he did earlier, when he was crawling through plastic tunnels in the office.

Figure 10.13 (Tray 12, February 27)

On the same day, after Peter finished the previous sandplay picture and drew the labyrinth picture, he moved to a second sand tray and created an even more defined figure. This was a human with legs. It is a more developed version of a human than the previous figure and clearly conveys that he is developing an ego of his own. He now has two legs on which to stand. Before, even though he was trying to stand on his own, he didn't have a foundation to support himself.

Figure 10.14 (Tray 13, May 14)

It is important to note that the alchemical stages are not necessarily progressive or linear. One can see elements of various stages along the journey. This tray may seem to depict regressive movement. It is a tray that represents the sixth alchemical stage of *mortificatio*, or the stage of death and destruction.

As he selected sandplay miniatures, Peter said he wanted to make a graveyard. The alchemical stage of *mortificatio* involves themes of defeat, torture, mutilation, death, and rotting (see the dismembered hand). After the stage of *separatio* (which appeared in the previous two trays), there are often death images. *Separatio* is closely connected with *mortificatio*

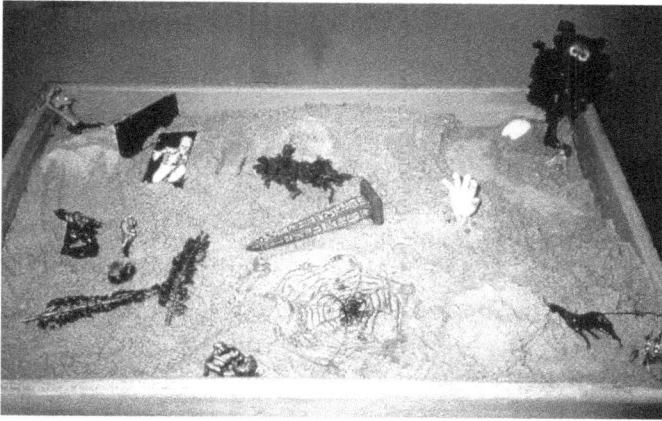

Figure 10.14 Tray 13

because *separatio*, or separation from the more familiar, is often experienced as a kind of death. It is likely that, when Peter began to experience himself as more independent, standing on his own two legs, there were feelings of loss. No longer could he feel the enmeshment of the previous younger relationship he had with his parents. This death is symbolized dramatically in this tray with the spider placed centrally in the graveyard.

Peter lit a gold candle and patiently let the wax drip over the mother spider enmeshed in her web. The spider is often but not always a symbol of the negative maternal and in this case that interpretation seemed to apply. This could be a death and funeral ritual, helping him to let go of his old relationship with his mother. In the sand, he placed a meaningful figure watching this ritual. It was Mowgli, the motherless child from *The Jungle Book*.

Peter's relationship with his mother in his outer world was going through a profound change. On this same day, his mother complained that Peter was angrier at home than ever before. At the same time, not so surprisingly, he was doing beautifully in school. The same process in the tray was happening at home, i.e., destruction and death of the old Peter and an attempt to find the stronger independent legs he needed. Yet, his volatile emotions were, at times, getting out of control. The therapeutic intervention at this time was to teach him a way of understanding and verbalizing his anger in a more positive acceptable way than merely acting it out. I hoped that learning a conscious way to express anger, along with continued involvement in the powerful sandplay process, would lead him in a new and creative direction. Therefore in therapy, we discussed anger and appropriate ways to express it. Here again in a tray – now up front and next to Peter – is the golden-colored primitive person, mixing something in a cauldron.

Figures 10.15 and 10.16 (Tray 14, Making the Gold, May 28)

This is Peter's last tray, created two weeks later. At Peter's request, a series of pictures was taken while he created this final tray. This tray went through a dramatic, evolving process. Peter knew that this event was a very special happening in the therapy work. The dynamic evolution of his final tray reveals a living illustration of unfolding psychic development, as seen from an alchemical perspective.

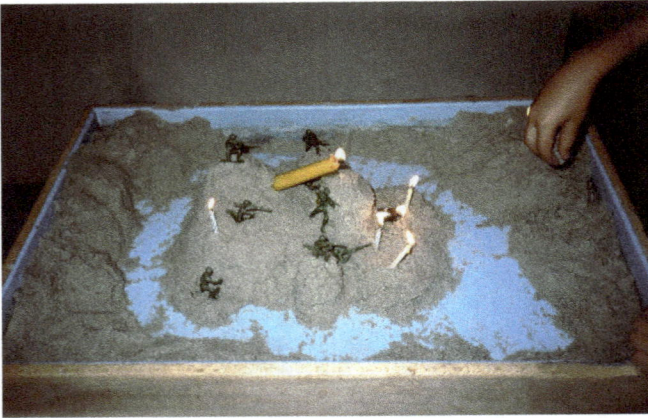

Figure 10.15 Tray 14, Making the Gold

If I were to try to fantasize what type of process would best illustrate the connection between sandplay and the alchemical process, I couldn't have come close to what really happened. It surprised and amazed me. I felt in awe about the way the unconscious moves and is demonstrated so graphically in these scenes.

Peter created this tray using six basic elements or stages of the alchemical process: (1) water, represented by the blue of the tray and his choice of wet sand, suggests the stage of *solutio*; (2) the separation of the island from the rest of the land represents the stage of *separatio*; (3) the melted wax of the candles represents the stage of *coagulatio*; (4) the fire of the lighted candles represents the *calcinatio* stage; (5) the smoke from the candles, *sublimatio* (divert or modify into a culturally higher or socially more acceptable activity); and (6) *mortificatio* is represented by the dead soldiers.

When this tray was in its earliest stage, it seemed unlikely that he would be able to bring all these elements together to reach a higher level. That highest level, according to alchemical thinking, is *coniunctio* – a perfect joining of all elements resulting in the creation of gold, which is the goal of the alchemical process.

Then, Peter felt both the wet and dry trays and settled on the wet one. In the middle of the tray, he created a flat-topped island with a hole in the middle for a candle. He deliberately placed the large lighted candle sideways, so that it would drip onto the sand. Then, he placed five lighted birthday candles around the tray. Next, he selected another large candle, which he cantilevered over the original big candle. The original candle can't be seen in the picture; it is hidden by the sand mountain. Next, he carefully placed the dead and dying army men, sculpting the island as he went, finding the perfect place for each of the men. He then asked the therapist to take a picture.

Immediately afterward, he asked to turn off the lights, and he and the therapist silently watched in the darkness for a long time as the candles burned down and listened to the music of the crackling sound of hot wax hitting the wet sand. What a dramatic event this was. He then asked to have a second picture taken, **Figure 10.16**.

Possibly, this process of experiencing and re-experiencing and then confronting his own darkness with the light was an important element in giving him the ego strength he needed.

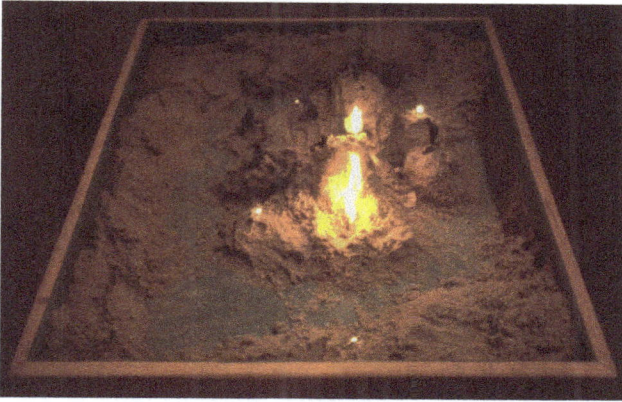

Figure 10.16 Tray 14, continued

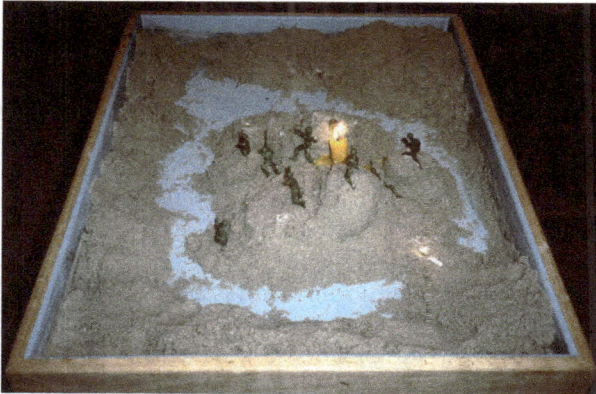

Figure 10.17 Tray 14, continued

Figure 10.17

With the birthday candles almost extinguished, Peter then raised the central candle to shed light on the tray and serve as a marker in this graveyard of dead soldiers. For transformation or growth to occur, one must be able to work with and shed light on dark feelings.

He then took the central candle and put it on its side, thus, uncovering the second large candle that was almost buried in the sand. In unearthing the second candle, he discovered with delight that the two yellow candles had left a considerable residue of molten wax in the sand. This discovery seemed to intensify his efforts and he became even more focused and determined, as though he, as an ancient alchemist, was working passionately in his laboratory.

Figure 10.18

With the fire out, the wax from the two candles flowed together, and a new meaningful symbolic form emerged. The opposing forces within him were leading him to the development of something new, yet he did not seem satisfied.

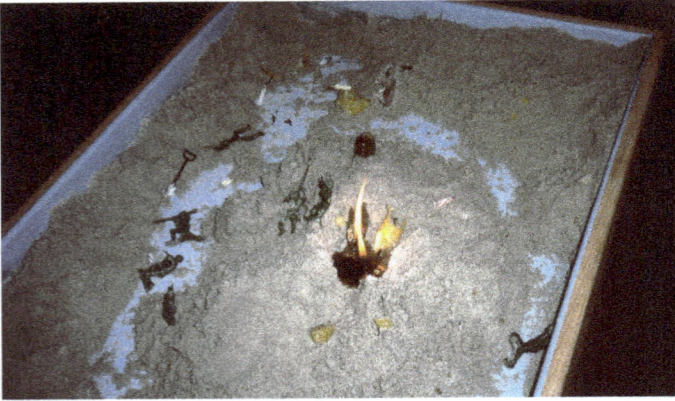

Figure 10.18 Tray 14, continued

He then proceeded to light a match and ignite the remaining wax. Obviously, there was more to be cooked – the transformation was not yet complete (Traditionally, alchemists used two firing processes). Now, there were two flames burning from the lighting of one match. Eventually, the two flames became one flame. Peter then completely focused on the center of the tray. At this stage, he removed the dead army men and the residue of the birthday candles from the tray. We watched again as the single flame burned down.

Figure 10.19

From wet sand and heated wax, his process created a spherical vessel of golden wax. How proud he was as he stepped back and viewed the scene, even though he didn't have a conscious awareness of all that he had done. With this process of *coniunctio*, the final stage of the alchemical process had been completed, and the goal of the opus had been achieved. He had created gold!

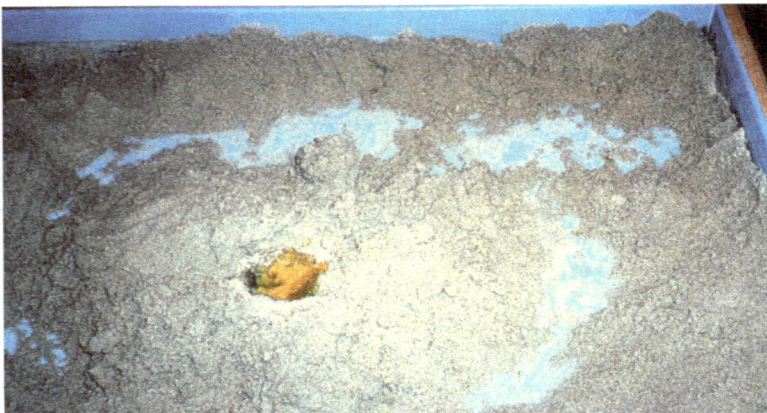

Figure 10.19 Tray 14, continued

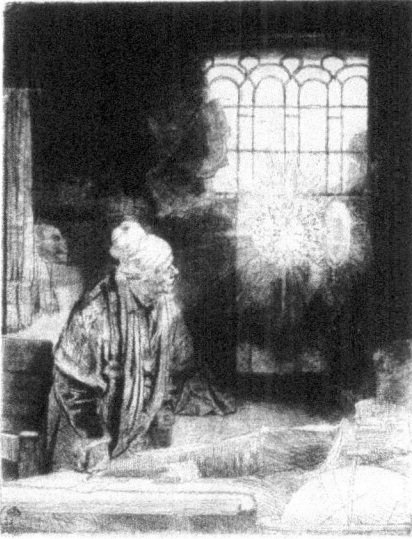

Figure 10.20 Drawing of an aged alchemist

Epilogue

Peter continued in therapy for about two more months. During this time, he seemed to settle down even more. His mother reported that he seemed less irritable at home and more focused in school. The last time his mother made contact with me was about three years later, right after the Northridge earthquake in 1994. She said that, although their house had been hit quite hard, Peter and his sister were not showing signs of stress at that point. She wanted some ideas about how to deal with them in the future, if they did begin to show anxiety. She said that Peter was doing well in school and that he was playing soccer.

To conclude, please view **Figure 10.20** – a famous Rembrandt drawing of an aged alchemist dressed in his long, flowing robes, working in his European laboratory over 300 years ago. Then, while holding this image in your mind, imagine eight-year-old Peter, dressed in his long T-shirt (that reached almost to his knees), his baggy pants, and Nike shoes, working in his own laboratory – the sand tray – during the present time in Los Angeles. For Peter and for this ancient alchemist, the time and place could hardly be more different, but the process was the same.

References

Edinger, E.F. (1985). *Anatomy of the psyche: Alchemical symbolism in psychotherapy*. Ingram Book Company. (Reprinted 1999 by Open Court Publishing Co.).

Jung, C.G. (1968). *The collected works of C. G. Jung: Psychology and alchemy* (Vol. 12). Princeton University Press. (Originally published 1944).

Kalff, D. (1980). *Sandplay: A psychotherapeutic approach to the psyche* (W. Ackerman, Trans.). Sigo Press.

Chapter 11

Combining play therapy and sandplay therapy

This chapter discusses the use of sandplay therapy within a play therapy context. Both play therapy and sandplay therapy provide children with the opportunity to use symbolic objects to communicate their thoughts, feelings, fantasies, and experiences nonverbally to an accepting and supportive therapist. While both play therapy and sandplay therapy can serve as a window into a child's internal world, sandplay adds structure to relatively unstructured play therapy, while play therapy provides a wide range of activities. Typically, a flexible combination of play therapy and sandplay therapy, plus appropriate talk therapy, is used, guided by the preferences of the child client.

For most children, play therapy is the only way to express and communicate their difficulties; often it is not until adolescence that words are used in therapy to express inner issues. Both play therapy and sandplay therapy provide children with the opportunity to use symbols to express feelings and difficulties nonverbally.

When a child enters the "free and protected space" (Kalff, 1980) of a playroom that contains a variety of small and large toys, sand, and other play equipment, the child's imagination is immediately stimulated, and the natural healing powers of the psyche are enlivened, allowing the child to express and "play through" the issues that have brought him or her to treatment. The space is considered to be "free" because children can create whatever they desire in the sand and "protected" because the therapist is present to protect the child and space from intrusions, harm, and other distracting events. The presence of the therapist who understands the literal and symbolic meaning of the toys supports positive development and growth of the child through either silently witnessing the creation of a sand picture or actively playing with the child during play therapy.

Therapeutic play

Although most children are naturally drawn to the toys in a playroom, many child therapists have found that an introduction to the playroom and toys facilitates and sets the tone for therapeutic play. Some therapists, for example, introduce the playroom by saying (with an "awe-inspired" voice) while motioning to the room and toys, "This is a very special place where you can play and do almost anything you like here." Some add, "I will tell you if you can't do something." Thus, the child knows that there are some limits in the room. Typical limits are developmentally appropriate rules, such as not hurting oneself or others, inappropriate destroying of property, etc. The therapist may then suggest that the child look or walk around the room to choose what would be fun to do.

When introducing sandplay, directions are somewhat more specific than in introducing play therapy. Sandplay therapists often say, "Here are two trays filled with sand. As you can see, one tray is wet; the other tray is dry. Would you like to feel the sand?" Then, "Here (gesturing to shelves of miniatures) are small, miniature toys and other objects you can use in the sand trays. If you like, you can use these objects to make a picture in the sand." Later, if the client does create a sand picture, sandplay therapists often add, "After you leave today, I am going to take a picture of what you've made in the sand, if that is all right with you, so you can later see all of your sandplay pictures." Usually children are uninterested in seeing pictures of their "old" sandplay trays; they are busy creating new aspects of their lives. However, a number of child clients return as adults to review their sandplay worlds.

Some therapists prefer a more organic introduction to sandplay therapy. They wait to see how the child intuitively uses the sand, water, and miniatures. If a child is playing with only the sand or the miniatures, the therapist may mention that the miniatures and sand can be used together to create a picture in the sand. Sandplay therapy, within the context of play therapy, allows a child to create an imaginative world by placing miniatures in a tray. Dora Kalff (1971), founder of sandplay therapy, said that sand represents instinct, nature, and the healing power of Mother Earth. Miniatures on nearby shelves are a stimulus to the child's imagination and represent many aspects in the child's world. A child's choice of miniatures helps the therapist to understand the issues that are displayed symbolically in the sand.

Thus, sandplay serves as a window into the client's inner world, and provides the opportunity to express a myriad of feelings, unspoken thoughts, and even the unknown. Sandplay scenes may be created quickly, in as little as ten minutes, or take the entire therapeutic hour. Usually, a sandplay picture is not created at every therapy session; it is the child or adult client's choice when, and if, to use sandplay.

After giving the child an opportunity to examine the toys and miniatures during the first session, some therapists ask, "Would you like to make a picture in the sand now?" The reason for inviting the child to create a sand picture during the first or second therapy session is that playing in the sand will often help the child feel more comfortable in the new environment. In addition, the content of the tray and the process the child uses in creating a sand picture can provide useful information about the child. For example, Kalff (1987) said that a first tray may suggest: (a) how the child feels about therapy; (b) the child's relationship to the unconscious; (c) the nature of the problem; (d) the solution to the problem; and (e) in our experience, the first tray can also give information about the child's relationship to the therapist. Also, because children under eight years tend to create trays similar to other children of the same age, it is possible to acquire a deeper understanding of the child's developmental level from the child's first sandplay creation, especially if the tray deviates from the norm (Bowyer, 1970).

Sandplay in a play therapy setting

Sandplay is one of many expressive arts therapy interventions that a therapist can use within a play therapy environment. Both sandplay and play therapy are considered to be mostly nonverbal and nondirective creative techniques. However, children do seem to talk more during play therapy than sandplay therapy, probably because in play therapy the child and therapist have face-to-face interaction and often play together; relating and reacting to each other is an important part of play therapy. In contrast, the child using sandplay has the opportunity to connect to his/her own internal self without verbal involvement of the therapist. In sandplay, the focus is strictly on the relationship to oneself so that the sand pictures reflect what is happening in the child's inner world. Thus, children usually create sand pictures mostly in silence with the therapist sitting nearby, observing the child as he/she plays or creates a picture in the sand.

While both play therapy and sandplay therapy can serve as a window into a child's internal world, sandplay adds structure to the relatively unstructured play therapy environment. For example, in sandplay, children are allowed to create a picture within the confines of the sand tray using miniature toys that are usually not used in play therapy. In play therapy, the therapist typically does not suggest the nature or outcome of the play; children play freely with any item in the playroom, as long as they stay within the traditional limits of play therapy. Some children, especially young children under eight years of age, prefer to play freely in the sand and not make a picture.

After a play therapist actively engages with a child in play therapy, the child may decide to create a sandplay picture. At this point, the therapist normally changes his or her role from an active participant in the play to a silent observer of the child's sandplay process. This allows the child's own natural imagination to be the guide in creating sandplay pictures.

It is important for the therapist to realize that the developmental level of the child affects how he or she uses sand and miniatures. Bowyer's (1956) research on the influence of age on the scenes created in a sand tray indicates that young children (two to three years of age) usually demonstrate little or no focus; trays are chaotic and disorganized, and they typically use only a small portion of the tray. Sand is often dropped and thrown outside of the tray.

Bowyer also found that children four and five years old often use only a small portion of the tray; however, they sometimes move toys around the tray, while fighting, making noises, and speaking for the miniatures. The sand is mostly used for burying and unburying miniatures. A fixed picture in the sand is unusual for children under five years of age.

At ages six or seven, children normally begin to use the full space of the tray and expand their ability to control the way they create the tray, with transport (e.g., cars, trains) often being used. Children eight and nine years old use sand in a constructive way, creating roads, waterways, and buildings – most of the tray is used, and miniatures are arranged to represent action rather than having to move the miniatures around the tray. At 10 and 11 years old, children frequently show control in the tray by using fencing. The peak age for use of fences and signs in the tray is ten. By 12 years of age, sand pictures are often indistinguishable from those created by adults (Bowyer, 1956).

Role of the therapist

The therapist's role in sandplay is to establish a free and protected space in which children can relax and allow their internal state to be accessed and expressed. This experience is similar in feeling to Winnicott's (1965) description of play therapy, "being alone in the presence of the mother," who is present and accepting but not intrusive.

However, play therapists often participate in the child's play, supporting, mirroring, and sometimes modeling and encouraging play behavior (Green, 2012). In contrast, child therapists who are also sandplay therapists generally sit near the child but to one side as the tray is being created, often taking notes but not involved directly in the child's play in the sand. This close proximity can help establish trust and rapport beyond just verbal interaction, including an unconscious connection between client and therapist. When a safe space is provided by an empathetic therapist, the child can truly relax, access his or her imagination, and allow the internal world to be safely experienced and expressed in the tray.

It is important for a sandplay therapist to know how to tolerate silence and the uncertainty of not always consciously knowing what the child is communicating. Watching and listening without using words may be unfamiliar and difficult for some therapists; however, silence is important in sandplay. "Silent listening," while maintaining an attitude of openness and acceptance, helps create a safe and protected space that leads to spontaneous expression in the tray.

Through the process of playing in the sand, creating pictures using miniatures, and/or actively playing outside of the sand tray, children can experience psychological and cognitive changes. Play allows children to express themselves nonverbally, retrieve memories of early childhood experiences, as well as become calmer and more at peace. To illustrate this therapeutic process with children, David's work in play therapy and sandplay therapy is discussed below.

Case of David

The case of David illustrates the synergistic effect of using play and sandplay together. Through the use of both of these techniques, plus talk therapy as he matured, David was able to come to terms with his fears and move out into the world in a more self-assured, confident manner.

David began therapy when he was seven years and six months old, and in the second grade. During nearly four years of almost weekly therapy sessions, he created a series of 25 sandplay scenes and participated in many play therapy activities. Some of these activities are discussed along with six of his sandplay trays. During his time in therapy, David moved from an anxious, frightened child to a more relaxed and confident preteen.

My first impression of David was of a skinny, frail-looking wisp of a boy. He seemed so anxious, helpless, and depressed that my first impulse, which I had to control, was to reach out and take care of this weak and lethargic child. Although David was normally silent at home, in his first session he talked openly about his experiences and feelings, and from the very beginning he was very committed to attending therapy sessions regularly.

Initially I did not know that his fears and fantasies had entrapped his life energy; thus, his energy was unavailable to him to use in his outer life of school and relationships. Early on, he told me that he felt different from others in many ways.

Background information

Before David started therapy, I met with his mother; his father was unable to attend this session. She reported that David's symptoms included stomach cramps, which appeared during school months but disappeared during vacation. He also had sleep problems since birth, including insomnia, sleep terrors, and sleep walking. When he was stressed, he had strong emotional reactions, including rage, tears, and once, when he was six years old, a threat of suicide. Additional symptoms concerned his mother: thumb-sucking at home but not at school; excluding himself from social contact with peers (even when his peers wanted to be with him); unfocused speech patterns; and underachievement at school, including not finishing his work and daydreaming. His mother commented, "The impression is that David is slow, but actually he is bright. I have a bright boy who doesn't know how to communicate it to the world."

David is a middle child with two sisters. His older sister, an intellectually gifted teenager, was actively involved with friends and extracurricular interests. His younger sister was born about 18 months after David. His mother thought that perhaps David was not given as much attention as he needed, since their births were so close together. However, she said that she feels a very special connection to David, and she is much more protective of him than she is of her daughters.

David's father is a police officer. David's mother described her husband as having a "horrible temper." She said, "He gets angry unexpectedly, especially at David. My husband is not physically abusive, but when he gets angry and yells, it's as though he hates us. Most of the time, he worships the children."

The extreme worry that David's mother carried began even before his birth when the results of an ultrasound test suggested that David was missing one leg. At his birth, he was immediately taken away from her without reassuring comments from the doctor. While waiting to see her newborn son, her fears magnified and grew to incredible heights. Later, when David was finally brought to her, the doctor said, with apparent relief, "He's fine, just fine." However, the doctor's words and David's normal appearance did not relieve the terror she felt, and she continued to carry her fears when interacting with David.

Another important dynamic in understanding David's issues is that he had a very sensitive and intuitive nature, which left him with few defenses against the highly charged issues in the home and in his inner and outer worlds. For example, David was described by his mother as "very perceptive." According to her, if David said something was going to happen, it would happen or had already happened. She cited this example: one evening, his policeman father was on a stakeout, waiting for suspects in a burglary to appear so he could arrest them. At home, without any knowledge of what his father was doing, David suddenly became very upset and told his mother, "Dad is chasing some criminals, and they pointed a gun at him." Later, when she told her husband what David had said, he verified that David's description of the arrest was correct. His mother told me that this type of knowledge was typical for David, and he intuited happenings in other situations as well, not just with his father.

I came to realize that David's withdrawn and inhibited behavior was supported by a whole spectrum of difficulties: (a) his mother's anxiety and fear for him, which resulted in her becoming over-protective; (b) his father's anger and rejection of David because of his timidity, which made David feel even more frightened, worthless, and helpless. David's own sensitive nature both caused, and was a result of, his intuitive and close connection to his mother and his father's angry and negative behavior toward him.

Therapeutic process

During our first therapy session together, David best expressed his view of the family dynamics when he drew a picture of his family doing something (a kinetic DAP). It showed four of his family members riding in a motor boat, looking straight ahead, while the boat pulled David along behind on water skis. No one was paying attention to him. David did feel very much alone, although his being alone was largely due to his own choice.

One of David's favorite activities in play therapy was to "play fight," with each of us holding a *Bataka* (i.e., a heavily padded paper cylinder with a handle at the end). In addition to "fighting," David enjoyed trying to knock my *Bataka* out of my hands while I tightly grasped it length-wise between my hands. When he was able to hit it hard enough so it flew out of my hands, he would laugh with glee and pump his muscles. He also enjoyed playing board games, especially when he won, and he loved playing with puppets; they could express what he could not.

Later in therapy, we explored the stream and small hills outside of my office. We even played a little soccer and baseball, although he soon found out that I was no challenge. Mainly, toward the end of therapy, we talked about his life, the challenges he experienced with his father, the demands of his school work, and his growing enthusiasm and abilities in athletics. Throughout his therapy he created sandplay pictures, which not only chronicled his growth and development but also allowed him to express what was happening consciously and unconsciously in his life.

During his therapeutic process, David created 25 sandplay scenes from the age of 7.5 to just past 12. The sandplay scenes represent various aspects of his development during his nearly five years in therapy. David named all of his sandplay scenes, which is unusual for a child his age. Six of the scenes are discussed below. For each sandplay picture, the following information is given: David's name for the sandplay, David's age, and the number of the sandplay in his series of 25 trays.

Figure 11.1 (Tray 1, age 7.5, "MASH Unit")

In the center of the sand tray, David placed a bandaged man on a stretcher, with two doctors, a male and female, standing on each side of the stretcher. David moved the sand so that these miniatures appear contained within a womb-like space. Nearby and to the right is an ambulance. Above the stretcher and slightly to the left are three objects that form a triangle: a spider, rock, and autumn tree. Four green trees surround the medical scene.

David's situation is depicted clearly in this tray, suggesting a strong (and perhaps porous) connection to the unconscious. The tray has a somewhat barren and empty quality; its starkness suggests isolation, desolation, and suffering, which is what David was experiencing at both home and school. His trays have an empty quality, depict injury, and contain prone figures, suggesting the possibility of early wounding.

The prone, bandaged man on the stretcher is similar to David, wounded and helpless, both caught between his parents and needing their assistance. Help is available in the form of two doctors (male and female) and the ambulance. I noted that David placed the doctors and ambulance near to where I was sitting and where David was standing as he created his tray.

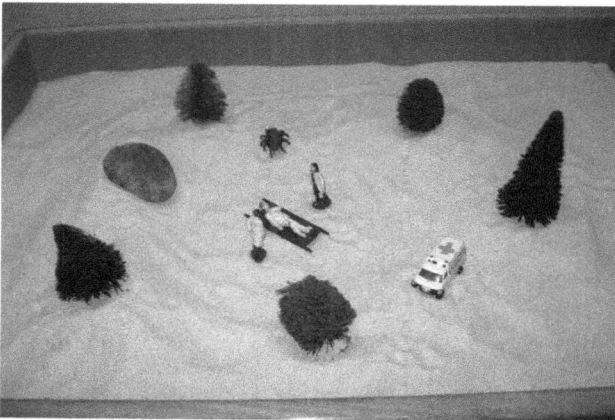

Figure 11.1 Tray 1, age 7.5

The spider, located above the wounded man, suggests potential for further wounding. The spider is most often viewed symbolically as a poisonous mother symbol. In David's outer life, he was caught in his mother's overanxious web of worry about his well-being. I believe her constant uneasiness and overprotective behavior was experienced by David as being caught and held back.

As I viewed the tray, additional questions came to mind: What do the four trees in the scene symbolize? Natural energy and growth? Or, perhaps they represent the four other people in his family? Do the ambulance and doctors placed near to us indicate a positive transference and that perhaps help is now available?

The dying evergreen tree at the back of tray concerned me, as did the rock and the spider, which seemed to be threatening the wounded man. I wondered about David's potential to resist change and growth in therapy. I hoped that the four green and vibrant trees represented David's life force and would help him connect to the energy he needed to move forward.

Figure 11.2 (Tray 2, age 7.6, The Big Parade)

In this tray, help is again available. The same wounded man (from the first tray) is now in a jeep (left/middle) with the doctor and nurse. Presumably, he is being taken to a hospital for treatment. The parade (representing David's psychological movement), includes a horse-drawn gold coach, which is being protected by the police and soldiers from intrusion by the bicycle riders and the black spider (behind the doctors in the jeep).

Work machines (a cement mixer, dump truck, and tractor) suggest that internal work is going on. I was pleased to see that David placed a white shell in the midst of the parade (near the middle, front of the tray). The shell is one of the eight emblems of good luck in Chinese Buddhism, signifying a prosperous journey.

With the alligator and spider penned (top/left), I could see that David was now in the process of containing elements that may have hindered his development in the past. The alligator and spider are considered symbols of negative archetypal maternal energies (alligators feed only their babies who snap at flies; spiders eat their young). The snow-covered wintergreen

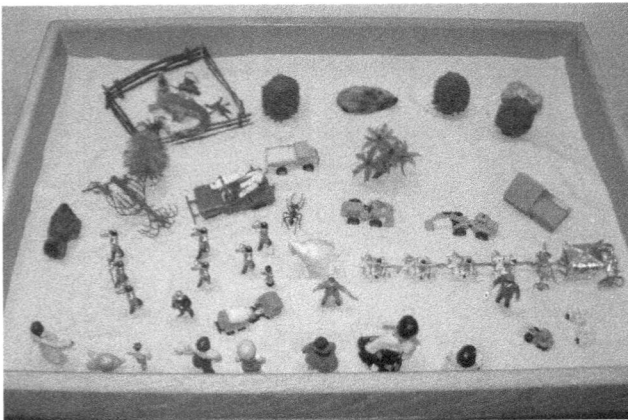

Figure 11.2 Tray 2, age 7.6

trees suggest that growth and development are possible, but the trees are currently dormant; thus, change may not happen immediately. The rock from his initial tray (top/right corner) and the driftwood (middle/left) also suggest that change may be slow (i.e., rocks and driftwood take time to form and change). However, the four small palm trees nestled together near the top/middle of the tray suggest the possibility of growth and development even in the most difficult of circumstances, for palm trees are strong and highly resilient.

I was happy with this tray, because I always hope to see movement in a second tray suggesting that the psyche is beginning to shift and possibly change in a positive way. However, the rock and driftwood reminded me that, while progressive elements (the parade and trees) are alive and active in David's process, regressive and resistant aspects are also evident in this tray; the rock suggests resistance and inflexibility. Now, as I look back on this tray, I see that the natural piece of driftwood symbolized David's therapeutic process (i.e., that transformation would occur but through a natural process that would take some time).

Figure 11.3 (Tray 8, age 9.0, Testing the Animals)

About one-and-a-half years later, David created this tray. He was doing somewhat better in school, and he was a member of a Little League baseball team. In this scene, David placed two males and a female (he called them "scientists") in front of enclosures that housed untamed animals. David said that the scientists were studying the animals' behavior.

The scientists in the sand tray suggest that it was now possible for David to have the ability to think about and develop a more objective attitude about his situation. The primitive and younger aspects of his psyche – the alligators, giraffe, lions, and bear (in the cage on wheels, located on the right side of the tray) – are now separated. This is a necessary separation if David is to disentangle himself from his enmeshed family.

It may be possible for the lion to escape from its cage through the break in the fence. If this "break" were to happen for David, it would then be possible that David's wild, primitive energies could either overwhelm him or bring him the considerable primitive strength he needs.

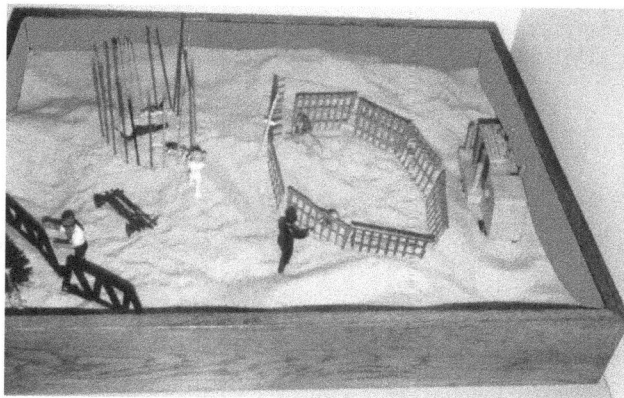

Figure 11.3 Tray 8, age 9.0

A giraffe, on the left-front side of the tray is eating, taking in nourishment. As the tallest species, a giraffe has a wide range of vision and symbolizes objectivity of thought. Objectivity is necessary in David's life, helping him rise above his family situation of both overprotection and rejection.

Almost immediately after David made this sand tray, his behavior and sand trays moved in a new direction. Now, with clearer vision and an objective ego, David took a more differentiated stance. He seemed better able to use his fine mind, which aided him in his task of separation and individuation and freed him to embark on his necessary hero's journey, as well as integrate his stronger, more positive capacities in his everyday life.

Figure 11.4 (Tray 12, age 10.1, Babies Take Over)

After smoothing the sand, he randomly placed the babies, with two of them sitting on a jet plane. He positioned rifles beside some of the babies. Next, David lined soldiers along the front of the tray with their hands up in the air, facing the babies as if they were surrendering.

As David drew barely visible lines in the sand, linking the men to the babies, he told me that the lines were electric wires, which the babies could pull and electrocute the men if they moved. He said, "The babies are tired of being bossed around. They have become bad now. Their pictures are on the 'Most Wanted' posters, so the guys have come after them."

I was pleased to see that David was displaying so much new energy (the babies). However, many questions came to my mind as I reflected on the tray, and I wondered what had been awakened in David. Perhaps he had discovered new independence and strength? If so, would this new power endanger his new energy (i.e., the babies)? I also gave some consideration to the possibility that this was a regressive tray. However, I was more convinced that David was finally gathering his strength to deal with the destructive masculine energy in his home.

Around this time, at ten years of age, David was willing to discuss his relationship with his father in more detail than ever before. He told me about his father's unpredictable temper, and how scared he felt when he was younger. Now, he found he could relate to his father through sports. They both enjoyed watching sporting events together on television. He seemed to be

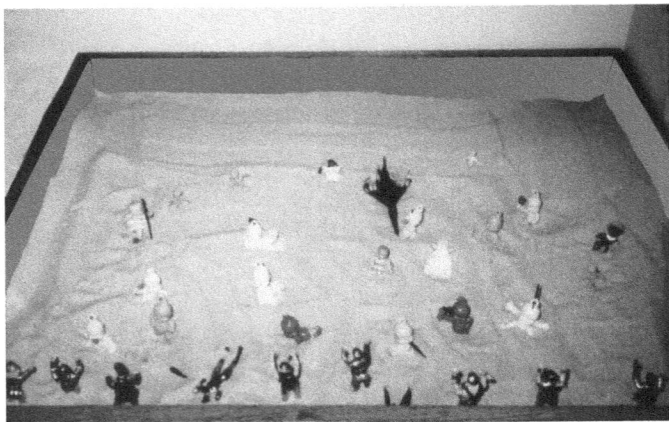

Figure 11.4 Tray 12, age 10.1

gathering strength despite his mother's overprotectiveness. However, the babies in the tray suggested that this energy was still very new, quite young, and undeveloped. I knew that he would continue to need support in his development.

In play therapy, David was spreading his wings and we often ventured outside of the office, taking walks, fording small streams, and climbing nearby hills. He shared with me his success in baseball; he was chosen the league's "Most Valuable Player." Around this time, he was also performing at a high academic level. His school identified him as "gifted," and he entered that program.

For many months David did not create sandplay scenes. Then, one day, he walked into the play room and immediately went right to work in the sand and made two trays.

Figure 11.5 (Tray 16, age 12.0, Fight for the Crown)

As David was making the tray, he told me the following story:

> These babies are in trouble. The Indians (upper/left and upper/right) are trying to steal their crown and candles (six white candles that he placed in the candelabra in the center of the tray, along with the crown). But the babies have a plan – if the bad guys get closer, the babies will take the candles and crown, and put them into the lifeboat. Then the babies will use their special powers and lift the lifeboat into the sky away from the bad guys.

The central organizing principle, the Self, is symbolized by the circular area that David carefully delineated in the middle of the tray. With this emergence, David now was able to display a stronger sense of self. Within this area, he placed the crown, candelabra, silver lifeboat, and four babies. Four is the number of wholeness. The lifeboat is a symbol of help, rescue, and safety. The candelabra, near the lifeboat, offers warmth, energy, light, and consciousness to the situation. The crown is a visible sign of success and of "crowning" achievement.

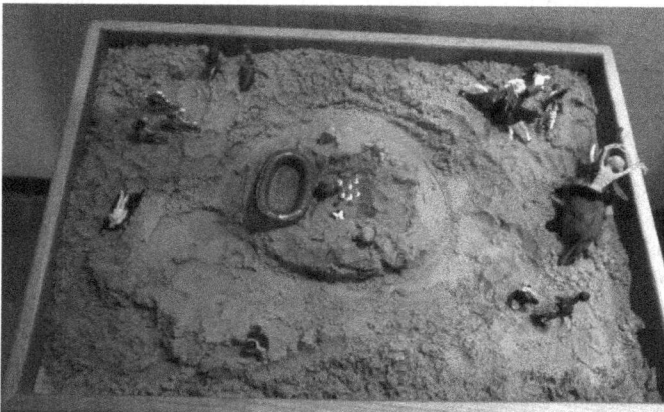

Figure 11.5 Tray 16, age 12.0

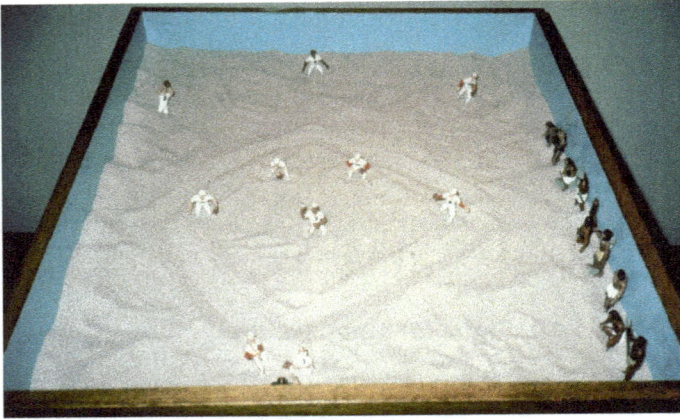

Figure 11.6 Tray 17, age 12.0

Despite the threatening and possibly destructive forces of the unconscious nearby (i.e., the Indians), David was now able to separate and protect himself from their potential invasion; the tortured figure on the elephant is leaving the tray and the wounded man takes a more distant position. He is aided by the four clever and imaginative babies, who represent newly emerging aspects of himself.

Figure 11.6 (Tray 17, age 12.0, The Baseball Game)

After completing the previous sandplay, David began to play with the sand in the second tray. I asked if he wanted to create another picture. He responded "yes." As he quickly made this tray, he explained that the two baseball teams have traveled through time and represent the best teams from their worlds.

In the symbol of the baseball diamond, it was clear to me that David's internal Self had at last become consolidated and connected to his ego (his outer life). Therefore, now both his inner and outer worlds are more connected. I watched with pleasure as David quickly and with confidence placed a baseball team on the diamond he outlined in the sand. The diamond shape is a powerful symbol of the totality of the Self. Through the game of baseball on a diamond shaped field, David has now found an age-appropriate connection to the outer world. The opposing team of cave men, waiting on the sidelines, symbolized the archaic, primitive, and archetypal aspects of David. In the past, these aspects had attempted to take over as well as detract and pull him in a regressive direction, often successfully. I was pleased to see that the cave men were now on the sidelines.

Conclusion

After David's seventeenth sandplay, he continued in therapy for quite a while, using the time to paint, play games, and talk. He created eight more sand trays, which suggested further consolidation and strengthening of his independence and ego. With his newfound awareness,

David then worked in conjoint therapy with one of his sisters to deal with their family concerns. He was performing very well in school when he terminated therapy.

I last heard about David when he was 14 years old and in the eighth grade. He was successfully involved in baseball and football. That year he won the league's "Most Valuable Player" award in football, and he was chosen for the US youth baseball team scheduled to go to Beijing, China, that summer. He was liked and respected by his teachers and was popular with his peers, although he still enjoyed being alone and did not socialize easily with others.

David's mother now described him as a quiet person who is calm and consistent under the pressure of sports. She believed that he was particularly astute in understanding and meeting his own needs. For example, he decided not to participate in basketball that year (even though he also excelled in that sport) because he needed leisure time between the busy football and baseball seasons.

It appears that, as a teenager, David was able to access his own inner strength, while his outer life was a natural reflection of his own distinctive abilities and interests. As he further matures, there will be more room for his excellent intellectual abilities to emerge. Whatever his future, I am certain that David will live it in his own unique way.

References

Bowyer, L.R. (1956). *Bulletin of British psychological society.* Summarized in L.R. Bowyer (1970), The Lowenfeld *world technique*. Pergamon Press.

Green, E.J. (2012). The Narcissus myth, resplendent reflections, and self-healing: A contemporary Jungian perspective on counseling high-functioning autistic children. In L. Gallo-Lopez, & L. Rubin (Eds.), *Play based interventions for children and adolescents with autism spectrum disorders* (pp. 177–192). Routledge.

Kalff, D.M. (1971). *Sandplay: Mirror of a child's psyche.* The Browser Press.

Kalff, D.M. (1980). *Sandplay: A psychotherapeutic approach to the psyche* (W. Ackerman, Trans.). Sigo Press.

Kalff, D.M. (1987). *Sandplay with Dora Kalff.* (Seminar notes). University of California at Santa Cruz.

Winnicott, D.W. (1965). *The family and individual development.* Tavistock Publications.

Chapter 12

Sandplay with adults

Sandplay is a widespread and conventional form of therapy for children. Using sandplay with adults, who possess conceptual language, is less conventional. However, language only partially succeeds in conveying intensely felt emotions, affects, and tensions that even adult clients are often unable to express, control, or understand. Sandplay offers an avenue to reach and communicate with these inner experiences, as well as heal deeply buried wounds.

With adults, sandplay can offer an opportunity to play creatively and express oneself spontaneously, without words, often for the first time since childhood. Through the free experience of play, the cognitive-logical mind is put aside, and the innocent, unsophisticated, and unconscious elements of the psyche, heretofore repressed, are allowed to emerge.

Once these elements are made available, healing energies can be released to help the individual perceive and deal with life issues. Through this experience, unrealized aspects of the personality can be discovered, made conscious, and integrated, leading to a sense of greater balance and wholeness and an enriched, more satisfying life.

Chapter 8 discusses many of the differences between the sandplay creations of children and adults. This chapter presents special considerations that are important in using sandplay with adults.

Some characteristics for all ages

A basic premise of sandplay therapy, in the Jungian tradition, is that the psyche possesses a natural tendency to heal itself, given the proper conditions. Similar to how our physical wounds heal under beneficial conditions, the psyche also has an instinctual wisdom that emerges when left free to operate naturally in a protected environment. Using miniatures and the sand tray, and through the experience of free and creative play, unconscious processes are made visible in this three-dimensional form, much like a dream experience. Thus, sandplay provides a vehicle for the unconscious to let itself be seen and known.

The most important aspect of using this technique is the preparation and personal development of the individual therapist. Estelle Weinrib (1983) speaks of the naïveté of some therapists who consider the addition of a sand tray to their practice:

> It would be an unfortunate misunderstanding to believe all one needs is a tray with some sand, a collection of small objects, and a dictionary of symbols. Just companioning a patient while s/he makes pictures will not accomplish much, nor will interpreting pictures as though they were dreams. (p.29).

Becoming an effective sandplay therapist is an engaging and circuitous process that requires the ability to receive, facilitate, and understand the profound experiences and symbolic imagery that this medium can evoke. Comprehensive clinical training, involvement in one's own personal therapy, and experience as a practicing therapist are all important. It is recommended that therapists interested in sandplay training read and take courses in sandplay, Jungian theory, and symbolism, and complete their own sandplay series to enhance understanding of the therapeutic process as it unfolds in this particular medium. A sandplay consultation group experience can be helpful. To the extent that therapists have experienced and found meaning in their own sandplay journeys, they will be able to grasp the meaning and implications of their clients' sand trays.

Although the sandplay process may appear to be straightforward, and even simple, the complexities of the approach soon become apparent. Most important is the presence of a therapist who values the healing powers of the unconscious and is able to provide a safe space for the client.

The role of the sandplay therapist is to establish a *free and protected space* in which the client can relax and let his or her internal state be accessed and expressed. This free and protected experience is similar in feeling to what Winnicott (1965) describes as "being alone in the presence of the mother": in the sandplay session, the client has to be able to trust the process in order to allow connection with and to express his or her inner world, which eventually leads to contact with the inner self (i.e., the ground of a person's own being).

Similar to the "good enough" mother who is present and accepting but not intrusive, most sandplay therapists sit a little behind the client and to one side, hardly seen (except out of the corner of the eye), yet their presence is essential. This procedure helps to establish trust and rapport beyond verbal interaction, including an unconscious connection between client and therapist. When this space can be provided, the client can truly relax and access his or her imagination, so that the internal world can be experienced safely.

Introducing adult clients to sandplay

Over time and with experience, sandplay therapists evolve their own personal style of introduction. However, most sandplay therapists agree on three basic principles:

- The introduction should communicate a respect for the sandplay process and its ability to access the healing powers of the unconscious. The therapist conveys this respect either verbally, through the initial explanation, and/or nonverbally by his or her ability to contain and hold this experience as it unfolds
- Therapists using sandplay also attempt to convey an open and nonjudgmental attitude, implying that whatever emerges in the tray is appropriate and acceptable – that there is no right or wrong way of doing sandplay
- Sandplay therapists convey, either verbally or nonverbally, that specific suggestions for sandplay themes do not come from the therapist. The therapist is nondirective; clients may create any type of picture in the sand

Adults often need encouragement to begin sandplay for they experience uncomfortable feelings when thinking about playing in the sand and are often fearful of what will be unexpectedly revealed in their trays. Adults who are dedicated to focused, cognitive approaches in their own lives may be particularly reticent and may even denigrate this type of nonverbal process.

Introducing the tray to adults involves listening to their concerns while observing their nonverbal communication. Encouraging the client to release his/her creative imagination to become a partner in the process often helps the adult client bridge his/her initial discomfort, making it possible to participate more freely in sandplay. Conveying to the client that sandplay is an opportunity to access otherwise inaccessible parts of himself or herself and to communicate something that cannot be expressed in words can be intriguing and often helps overcome reluctance.

Many sandplay therapists do not immediately suggest sandplay to adult clients. Instead, they first use traditional talk therapy, establish a strong therapeutic relationship, and wait until the time is right. Typically, the right time arrives when a client feels stuck, needs a deeper or creative experience, needs to know or understand something in a different way, needs to access early wounding experiences, or is particularly interested in connecting to the unconscious. Then the therapist might suggest that the adult client create a sand picture, by simply saying that sandplay provides an opportunity to move to a deeper level of understanding.

If the client agrees to try this new activity, the therapist invites him or her to touch and move the sand (to become grounded). At this point, the sand acts as a magnet and, before clients realize it, their hands are autonomously sifting the sand, making tunnels, shaping mountains, runways, and riverbeds. It is then suggested that the client leisurely look over the shelves of miniatures and select those figures that capture his or her attention and seem to be asking to be placed in the sand tray.

Accompanying the sandplayer

During sandplay, therapists most often take process notes and draw a rough sketch of the finished tray, with any changes noted. While taking notes the therapist needs to remain attuned to the sandplayer's verbal and nonverbal communications, as well as his or her own feelings during the session. Process notes typically include the following:

- The type of tray the client chooses (wet or dry sand)
- The manner in which the sand is touched or sculpted
- If water is added; how the miniatures are examined, selected, or not selected
- The order in which miniatures are selected and placed in the tray (particularly, the first and last miniatures)
- The location of miniatures in the tray
- Changes made
- Client's comments
- Therapist's impressions and feeling reactions
- Dialogue that occurs

During the creation of a sand picture, little verbal exchange happens between client and therapist other than the occasional comment about a miniature or a feeling generated by making the scene in the sand. The therapist may offer help in finding a particular miniature but normally acts as a silent witness, observing and recording the process until a recognizable point occurs and the sandplay process comes to a resting place. The client often announces that he/she has finished.

After a sand picture has been created, the therapist may inquire about the client's feelings in making the tray or personal responses to the tray itself. Sometimes the client is asked if the sand picture has a name; other times the therapist might observe the placement of a miniature. After the client leaves, the therapist photographs the tray and disassembles it out of the client's view.

In working with adults, there are moments in the *verbal* process when it may be therapeutically advisable to draw parallels between current life issues and the client's sandplay creations. For example, a therapist may remark, as the client is discussing a specific problem, "That reminds me of the witch you placed in your last sandplay tray." Threading the verbal and nonverbal together at the right moment can promote further understanding. Sensitively judging the right time to make this type of observation while not hindering the client's non-verbal, unconscious process is part of the art of sandplay therapy with adults.

The therapist does not interpret the tray to the client, nor does he or she suggest that the picture be changed in any way. Sandplay therapists believe that the sandplay picture is a "snapshot" of the psyche and/or unconscious. Just making the sandplay picture itself is therapeutic; verbal interpretation at the time is unnecessary. Giving directions or asking what is going to happen next in the tray would direct the process, take the experience out of the moment, emphasize the performance aspect, and put the therapist in the driver's seat – rather than letting the psyche freely move in its own individual direction.

It is essential that the sandplay process and the therapist are allied with and supportive of the healing energies of the Self, rather than the ego desires of the therapist or client. When the therapist moves into the cognitive realm too quickly by verbally analyzing the tray or gives directions to the client to move miniatures or create or amplify a particular scene, these are ego-driven activities that interfere with the client's internal process. These kinds of directions can occur in response to the therapist's anxiety that a miniature (representing an aspect of the client's psyche) is in jeopardy, discomfort with shadow material, or fear of the unknown. When the therapist does not trust the process and instead imposes his or her need to bypass difficult issues in favor of a momentarily cheerful resolution, the client's natural internal process is at risk of being compromised.

To facilitate the deepest transformation, the therapist must be willing to witness the perilous aspect of the client's journey, the "dark night of the soul," and assist emerging healing energies as well as support the client's endurance in meeting this challenge. True healing comes from within. It cannot be bestowed or imposed from without. Each individual's psyche is undergoing its own process of change.

Reflection on a series of trays

Additional steps can deepen the sandplay experience for adults. After the conclusion of a sandplay process (i.e., a series of trays), therapists often review all of the client's sandplay trays with the client at some mutually agreed upon date. Most adults are quite interested in viewing and reflecting on their work, and they benefit from moving this unconscious material to the conscious realm.

Timing of the review is important. Client and therapist must both feel ready to view the trays. Some therapists feel that pictures of the trays should not be viewed until years after therapy has ended (Bradway, 1994) because moving too quickly into an interpretive, cognitive realm may hinder the gradual unfolding of awareness and understanding of unconscious material that continues after therapy has ended. Other therapists do not wait as long, judging that some clients are ready to integrate unconscious material more quickly and that a timely review promotes increased consciousness and ego strength.

Clients are often deeply affected by viewing their sandplay series. Some cry when seeing their inner struggles portrayed and convey relief that they no longer feel enslaved by these old struggles. Others, moved by the creativity emanating from their unconscious, express delight and surprise. At some point during the viewing, almost everyone laughs at the way the unconscious portrayed his or her drama. Some therapists and clients find value in reviewing a series of scenes more than once, perhaps several times, each time yielding new insights.

Adult clients most likely to benefit from sandplay

Sandplay therapy is most effective for those clients who are open to using a nonverbal symbolic technique to explore personal aspects that may be unknown or obstructing their development. Many of these clients are seeking increased insight and meaning and need to heal early wounds that continue to derail their full functioning as adults. Clients who have difficulty expressing themselves verbally because they feel blocked or inarticulate about their deep feelings are often open to, and grateful for, the increased "vocabulary" sandplay affords them. Sandplay also works well when cultural differences need to be bridged, especially when the client's primary language is different from that of the therapist.

Several sandplay therapists have discussed the types of clients most likely to benefit from sandplay therapy. For example, both Weinrib (1989) and Ammann (1991) identified similar types of clients: (a) those who have sustained a preverbal injury, often because of a disturbance in the primary relationship with the mother or mother figures, which made it impossible for them to grow up with a healthy trust in the world or in their own life process; and (b) those who have a fundamentally healthy and stable ego but whose worldview is too narrow and one-sided. Perhaps they lack a clear sense of identity or feel restless or depressed, sensing that an expansion of consciousness is necessary. Confronting these issues and encountering the authentic self in the sand tray disrupts old patterns and creates movement toward psychic development and individuation.

Although these two types of clients can benefit from sandplay, we have found that not all clients who have these needs respond to sandplay therapy. Additional characteristics are helpful, including:

- Openness to the creative unconscious
- Genuine interest in change
- Courage to withstand the pain and discomfort demanded in going beyond the *persona* or social mask
- Willingness to take psychological risks to achieve another level of development
- Curiosity about verbally inexpressible life issues such as death, dying, abuse, or trauma
- Inclusive attitude toward dreams, spontaneous inner images, and synchronistic happenings
- Have the capacity to think symbolically
- Recognition of the existence of another dimension of reality beyond ego consciousness

Adult clients least likely to benefit from sandplay

Questions a therapist might think about when considering sandplay therapy with a particular client are:

* Are severely emotionally disturbed clients candidates for sandplay?
* Is the client overreacting to the miniature display?
* Does the content of the tray contraindicate its use?
* Is sandplay being used as an escape mechanism?
* Is sandplay an optimum technique for this client?

Creating a free and protected space is basic to the climate of this therapeutic method; therefore, sandplay should not be used with clients who seem uncomfortable with this technique. Clients communicate discomfort one way or another, through words or body language. This discomfort may be very subtle, perhaps displayed in an almost imperceptible movement away from the tray and/or the miniatures. Other times, the resistance may be clear and open, not at all subtle, with a refusal to even touch the sand. Such resistance can suggest that the client is not prepared to grapple with tensions, problems, and inner conflicts that may emerge when using this technique. Ultimately, the therapist has to trust the client about proceeding; sandplay should never be encouraged with adults who resist its use.

Sandplay seems to be most difficult for those clients whose belief system does not include a valuing of the unconscious, noncognitive mind. These individuals often do not appreciate the imagination, are quite concrete or literal-minded, and have an excessively mental attitude toward life and themselves. The sandplay materials may seem childish and unrealistic to them. They may even denigrate this approach. Accessing the symbolic world through a visual-tactile mode of expression is not appealing to them, and they may be unable to move beyond a literal level of awareness.

Are severely emotionally disturbed clients candidates for sandplay?

There has been an ongoing discussion regarding the usefulness of sandplay with severely disturbed clients, such as those diagnosed with schizophrenia, clinical depression, or borderline characteristics (Miller, 1979, p.157). Some therapists are concerned that providing an array of symbols might reinforce the client's chaotic and confused inner view of the world, rather than helping the client sort options and deal with practical issues in the everyday world. However, another view, expressed by Perry (1973), contends that expressing inner chaotic, negative energy is an important step in finding and activating natural and internal healing powers.

In examining this issue, Betsy Caprio (1989) studied the initial sand trays of 50 adult residents in a short-term psychiatric facility and found no evidence that would contraindicate the use of the sand tray with *stabilized* depressed and schizophrenic patients. In fact, just the opposite seemed to be true: these patients appreciated the color, variety, and creativity brought into their lives by their involvement in using sand tray equipment, and they did not become more disorganized or chaotic in their thinking.

Caprio's most striking finding was the absence of extraordinarily bizarre imagery in the sand trays of this group of hospitalized patients. Many of the sand trays contained few elements that depicted illness or the hospital. Instead, the trays gave clues for the direction of further treatment when they revealed the following:

- Traumatic experiences that had not been expressed verbally
- Developmental arrests, which gave therapists indications of where reparative work might begin
- Specific areas of strength

Although Caprio found no negative effects from using sandplay with these patients, the selection process did eliminate patients who were too distraught or violent to attend this activity. In addition, these hospitalized patients had more containment than those in out-patient settings. Some therapists have noted that miniatures and sandplay equipment could become dangerous objects when used by aggressive patients. Therefore, until further researched, no conclusion can be reached about the use of sand trays and miniatures with extremely disturbed patients.

Is the client overreacting to the miniature display?

Once in a while, a client may appear to be overwhelmed by the array of figures on the shelves. A client may either speak about this feeling by saying that it seems too much to take in ("I can't focus on anything") or simply be unable to proceed in the activity. This reaction suggests that too much of the unconscious realm has been stimulated. In this case, the therapist should note the indecision, elicit the client's feelings, and attempt to dialogue about these. Through this intervention, the client's feeling of being flooded by unconscious material would either subside and the sandplay activity would proceed or a decision would be made together that this session was not an optimum time to create sand pictures.

The content of the tray may alert the therapist to the possibility that the client is feeling overwhelmed by this activity. Although it seldom happens, sandplay can activate the unconscious in certain individuals to such an extent that it may be wise to stop, relax (perhaps use a deep breathing exercise), and then discuss the client's feelings.

Is sandplay being used as an escape mechanism?

A very few adults use sandplay as an avoidance or escape mechanism in order to use up the time and avoid having to deal with the reality of a face-to-face relationship with the therapist. In this situation, it is important that the therapist note the client's reluctance and perhaps gently express this observation to the client, saying something like "I have noticed that you are so involved in sandplay that there is little time for a face-to-face dialogue." From this comment, a discussion might ensue that brings light to the client's reluctance to talk with the therapist.

The bottom line is: therapists must trust their own intuitive clinical sense about whether the situation is becoming destructive and overwhelming or if an important process is unfolding. When in doubt, the therapist should immediately elicit the client's feelings about participating in sandplay as well as voice his or her own concerns as the therapist. Ideally, the decision to continue or stop sandplay will be a mutual one.

Understanding sandplay pictures: Finding meaning from it all

The sand tray can be viewed and considered from a number of different theoretical perspectives; however, most sandplay therapists consider the following:

- **Client's Personal Information:** The client's age, gender, socioeconomic status, racial and/or ethnic group, spiritual beliefs, motivation for creating a tray, and other demographic information can be helpful in understanding the trays
- **Creation of Sand Picture:** In order to have a full understanding of a sand picture, it is important to be aware of the client's process in creating the tray. For example, is it created quickly or slowly, with a great deal of thought or spontaneously, with fear or excitement, etc.
- **Content of the Tray:** The tray's content should be carefully followed and recorded (either through photographs and/or sketches), noting objects used and their symbolic meaning; placement of miniatures and position changes; movement of sand; and overall organization and content of the sand picture, including themes, stages, and phases, particularly those in an initial tray
- **Sandplay Series:** It is important to notice how clients' sand pictures evolve over time, including what symbols are used regularly and how their location in the tray has changed; how the themes have developed and changed; and variations in the organization of the scenes
- **Sandplay Story:** Some clients tell a story about the sand picture; others are stimulated by the picture and recall past or present events and feelings. Listening carefully to the symbolic content, emotional overtones, themes, and story resolution of the sandplay story gives further insight into the client's internal process
- **Therapist's Feeling Response:** When the therapist can listen to his or her own feeling response and be aware of spontaneous images, a deeper understanding of the client's process and the sand creation itself can emerge

Keeping these considerations in mind will help in understanding sandplay scenes of your clients; however, sand pictures can still be quite perplexing. We hope that the next sections will bring clarity to your work with adults and expand your understanding of their creations. Of course, even with increased insight, it is important to remember that much of the unconscious *is* and *will continue to be* a mystery.

Initial trays

All sandplay expressions are important; however, the initial scene is usually especially important. It could be likened to a topic sentence in a paragraph where the overall theme of the unfolding drama is stated. Gloria Avrech (1997) says that an initial sand tray scene is a reflection of the sandplayer's psyche, similar to a mirror reflecting an energy that comes from the client's deepest self. In creating an initial tray, the sandplayer might be saying, without realizing it,

> Here is a possible place for my personal myth. Here is some of what I struggle with, some of what is easy for me, some of what is hard. Here is what has happened to me and what I might become (p.53).

Initial trays have also been likened to initial dreams. Initial dreams are the first dreams that clients report to therapists. These dreams and initial trays are generally understood to result from similar psychological processes. However, there are significant differences; principally,

an awake, conscious ego is involved in the sandplay process (as in all forms of active imagination), whereas that is not the case in dreams. Indeed, a common problem in the sandplay
process is that the client might be *too* awake, rational, and analytical. The therapist using
sandplay should try to reduce the impact of the client's conscious ego by advising the client to relax his or her mind and body and to refrain from planning out a sand tray scene in
advance, unless there is a specific reason for doing so. If there is a specific reason, this reason
should be in the therapist's notes for future reference.

According to Dora Kalff (1988), an initial tray can indicate:

- The client's personal problem
- A possible solution
- His/her relation to the unconscious
- How the client feels about therapy

Kalff particularly emphasized the importance of including one's (the therapist's) initial feeling response to a tray in coming to an understanding of what is being communicated by the
client. She advised therapists to identify the feelings activated as the first step when viewing
any tray.

In addition to recognizing one's her own feelings, Friedman (1986) often asks herself
these questions when viewing an initial tray:

- Where are the energy spots?
- Where are the trouble spots?
- What kinds of groupings are apparent?
- What types of problems are indicated in the tray?
- Where are the sources of strength or help in the tray?
- What miniatures are placed near or close to where the therapist is sitting?

The first sand picture that a client creates may not be his or her *initial tray*. Estelle Weinrib
(1983) warns that a first tray may be just pretty, but that the second tray may authentically
connect to the unconscious. There is some controversy among practitioners concerning what
qualifies as an initial tray; no clear-cut definition has appeared in the literature. The therapist
must use intuition, knowledge, and judgment to decide if a tray qualifies as an initial one.
However, if a client uses his or her rational mind to consciously select figures for the purpose
of representing specific events or personal characteristics that the client wants the therapist to
note (sometimes called a *persona* tray), then this would not qualify as an initial tray.

Should this occur, the wise therapist accepts what the client offers and waits for another
tray. In our experience, deliberate, conscious trays continue for only a short time. Usually
with the second tray, the descent into the deeper realm of the psyche begins. It seems that if a
client has a good enough connection with the therapist and feels a sense of containment and
safety in the therapeutic relationship, it is then possible to be at ease and let the unconscious
speak in the sand.

Symbolism

As in all kinds of play, the symbolic process in sandplay is as natural as breathing and can act
as a bridge into the psychic realm. Play, which taps into creativity and imagination, releases

instinctive energy and leads naturally to the use of symbols. Words themselves are symbols, but it is easy to become enmeshed in and constrained by words, perhaps believing that words are the only way to communicate, thereby failing to make use of other symbols. Using a variety of symbols is necessary to express feelings, gain a larger perspective, and connect to the inner world – which leads to the healing experience.

Two general categories of symbols emerging in psychological work are: *Individuation* and *Transformation*. The first category relates to the individuation process, and includes symbols of such motifs as the Great Mother, the Child, the Wise Old Man, the Hero, the Shadow, the Maiden, and the Anima (in a male) or Animus (in a female). The second category is comprised of uniting symbols that represent the instinctual guiding center of the Self: the Mandala, the Circle, the Diamond, the Squared Circle, and the Sphere are a few of the forms that represent this psychic center.

Symbols, represented by miniatures in the sandplay process, can be used as tools of expression that enable clients to reveal unconscious aspects and subtleties of their inner thoughts and feelings that speech and gestures may fail to communicate. Because symbols connect clients to unknown aspects of themselves, they can also carry the potential for transformation and healing. Winnicott (1965) believed that symbols help access inner psychic reality. He saw them as transcending "external world phenomena and the phenomena of the individual person who is being looked at" (p.168).

Symbols are portrayals of psychic reality, pointing to something so deep and complex that it cannot be reduced to a simple verbal concept; their totality is beyond conscious grasp. Symbols are numinous indicators of a client's values and worldview. "Symbols speak for the inner, energy-laden pictures of the innate potentials of the human being" (Kalff, 1980, p.29). Although the ultimate meaning of a symbol can only be inferred and intuited only within limits, symbols can reintroduce individuals to unknown aspects of the Self and help them reconnect with unconscious parts of themselves. Symbols carry the potential for transformation and healing precisely because they cannot be reduced to concepts that are easily verbalized, categorized, and understood.

It is important to remember that no conscious understanding of symbols on the part of the client is needed in sandplay. The symbol points to some perception, understanding, or process that is beyond conscious comprehension. It does not matter whether or not the meaning of the symbol is understood by the conscious mind. It is more a matter of inner intuitive knowledge.

Creating a safe and protected space that intentionally encourages and supports clients in using and experiencing symbols can have at least two significant benefits. First, connecting with symbols that have personal significance for a client helps to generate insights, transformation, and eventual healing. Second, understanding the meaning of the symbols represented in the miniatures and sandplay scenes can help a therapist understand what the client is communicating, both consciously and unconsciously, which enables the therapist to be of greater help to the client.

Jung (1968) stated that symbols arise spontaneously from two sources: the unconscious (which instinctively produces symbols), and a person's own personal experience. Both of these sources are important when viewing sandplay scenes. The therapist needs to give his or her initial attention to what the symbol in the sandplay personally means to the client and not jump to generalizations about a particular symbol. In order to discover what may lie at the deeper levels in an individual's psyche, the meaning of a symbol must be understood in terms of the individual's own private symbolic language. Building on the client's personal associations, a symbol can then later be amplified by looking into mythological, religious, and folk tale representations of similar material. Making connections to myth, history, fantasy, imagination, drama, and poetry can be a part of giving meaning and depth to the process.

If the therapist is able to maintain a metaphorical attitude when following the symbolic process, then the client's issues, strengths, and the direction of the healing process can emerge with more clarity. It is most helpful when the therapist has gained a broad understanding of the language of the unconscious and is able to follow the process and help the client establish connections to his or her external life situation.

In actual practice, the therapist's knowledge of a miniature or symbol is not shared with a client before his or her sandplay process has been completed. Moving the experience into the cognitive realm prematurely may interfere with the intuitive and instinctual processes that activate healing energies. At times, adult clients do spontaneously share their associations or ideas about a particular miniature. This is important information; most sandplay therapists would include such a client's comment in their notes to consider both at that point in therapy and also later when preparing for review sessions after the sandplay process had been completed.

Themes in sandplay scenes

Because the symbolic language of the unconscious is baffling at times, therapists may feel frustrated and confused when attempting to decipher sandplay pictures. In order to better understand sandplay scenes, some years ago we began to study the sandplay journeys of our clients to determine if we could identify patterns or themes in their work. A *sandplay theme* is defined as a principal visual image or set of images in a sandplay picture. We decided to study the thematic approach because then our observations could be supported by research and also because it is an organic, non-diagnostic method that is congruent with the nonintrusive process of sandplay.

We have identified a group of themes that cluster naturally into one of two groups: (a) themes of wounding and (b) themes of healing or transformation. Themes of wounding appear most often in the first sandplay pictures of clients who are suffering from the effects of abuse, trauma, illness, loss, or death of a family member in their early development. Themes of positive transformation or healing are more prominent in early trays of clients who had either grown up in healthy, less traumatic environments or were in the latter phases of therapy and were moving in the direction of healing and health. For all clients, we found that trays usually contained more themes of wounding early in therapy; as therapy progressed, themes of healing and wholeness took a central place. Themes are discussed in more detail and illustrated with a case in Chapter 7.

Transference issues in the tray

Over time, Kalff's views on transference evolved to include the idea that the relationship between client and therapist is sometimes expressed directly in the tray. Recently, therapists have begun to examine trays methodically for indications of transference. It is important to notice the many other ways the process and pictures reflect or address the therapeutic relationship. The ways in which the client uses miniatures and participates in other aspects of the sandplay process are underlying clues about his or her relationship to the therapist as well as personal feelings about earlier relationships with significant others. These are discussed in Chapter 9, with case examples.

Key distinctions between sandplay with adults and children

While some therapists recognize that using sandplay with adults is different from its use with children (Friedman & Mitchell, 2001), others report few differences in their approach. In a 1979 workshop, Kalff (as cited in Miller, 1979) said that she did not distinguish between adults and children in her use of sandplay; in her perception, the underlying psychodynamic principles and process were the same, so she made no adjustments in the procedure. Other therapists report that adults use sandplay less frequently than children and that they (the therapists) engage in more "introducing, explaining, directing, questioning, associating, interpreting, and integrating" when working with adults (Miller, 1979, p.136).

Certainly adults are psychologically and physiologically more mature, sophisticated, and able to participate more consciously in their own treatments, yet they are also more rigid and stuck and less adaptable, except with concentrated effort over long periods of time. Children are usually more resilient, spontaneous, and plastic, gravitating to the sand more easily than adults, and they have the ability to change over a briefer period of time.

Although adults are typically less active, playful, and spontaneous than children, the number of adults who use sandplay is still substantial. In an international survey of therapists who use sandplay, Friedman and Mitchell (2001) found that most of their adult clients created at least one sand scene. Internationally certified sandplay therapists indicated that 80% to 90% of their adult clients used sandplay at least once, while 60% of adult clients of non-certified therapists used sandplay. Twenty years earlier, Miller (1979) conducted a similar survey; however, he found that only 45% of adult clients treated by sandplay therapists made a sand picture. The increasing use of sandplay by adults may be due to greater awareness and acceptance of nonverbal approaches; certainly the field of psychotherapy has become more inclusive of *feeling* and *doing* rather than just *thinking* and *saying* over the past 20 years. Overall, more children participate in sandplay than adults. However, because certified sandplay therapists work more with adults than children, naturally a larger number of their adult clients create sandplays.

Because sandplay is an adjunctive therapeutic technique, the amount of time spent using it varies tremendously; sand pictures are not necessarily created at every session. A few adult clients use sandplay regularly, especially those who are therapists themselves and want to experience their own sandplay process to use this medium effectively with clients. Nevertheless, a larger number of adult clients use sandplay only occasionally. Sometimes weeks and even months (more rarely) go by between the making of individual sand pictures. Miller (1979) found that trays were made by clients in approximately 38% of the sessions or every three to four therapy sessions on average. Recently surveyed sandplay therapists report similar periodic use by their adult clients. But even when only a few sand trays are made over years and viewed periodically, the scenes do not seem at all random; instead, they appear to be part of a continuous therapeutic process (Friedman & Mitchell, 2001). During periods when scenes are not made, therapy proceeds as usual and includes talking about everyday problems and their relationship to early wounding experiences and developing insight into interpersonal relations, dreams, and life issues, as well as participating in other play and expressive arts therapies.

Adult sand creations are usually unlike those of children. Adults tend to use a greater area of the tray, boundaries are more clearly defined, aggressive feelings are depicted symbolically rather than acted out, and verbal comments are made rather than moving or throwing figures. To express issues of control, adults use topographical features such as mountains and streams to unify scenes rather than fences or other literal structures of control, as do children (Bowyer, 1959). When adult trays deviate from these broad norms and seem more child-like, it may be an indication that the client experienced trauma during childhood. Age differences are discussed in more detail in Chapter 8.

The constructive use of sand (i.e., moving sand to make roads, waterways, and paths) seems to depend more on individual personality traits than on age. Bowyer (1959) found that the movement of sand by individuals over seven years old indicates an ability to use inner resources creatively to enlarge or restructure the tray and, symbolically, one's own world.

Adult cases

Several of the cases in other chapters illustrate how the healing process unfolds in adult clinical cases; see the cases of Anna in Chapter 5, Margarita in Chapter 6, and Tammy in Chapter 7. Each of these women made major life improvements through their sandplay processes.

Some final thoughts

Using sandplay with adults can provide them an opportunity to play creatively and express themselves spontaneously, without words, for the first time since they were children. Although many adults initially are reluctant to use sandplay, once they realize that it is an opportunity to access otherwise inaccessible parts of the self, and communicate issues that cannot be expressed in words, the reluctance usually disappears. As these elements are made available, healing energies can be released to help the adults perceive and deal with life issues.

In our experience, the self-healing properties of the psyche activated by sandplay can deepen therapeutic work with adults, allowing them to communicate in a nonverbal way that opens up a whole new world.

References

Ammann, R. (1991). *Healing and transformation in sandplay: Creative processes become visible* (W.P. Rainer, Trans.). Open Court Publishing. (Originally published in German as Hilende Bilder der Seele).

Avrech, G. (1997). Initial trays: Clues to the psyche. In B. Caprio (Ed.), *Sandplay: Coming of age*. Los Angeles Sandplay Association in association with the C.G. Jung Bookstore of Los Angeles.

Bowyer, L.R. (1959). The importance of sand in the World Technique: An experiment. *British Journal of Educational Psychology, 29*, 162–164.

Bradway, K. (1994). Sandplay is meant for healing. *Journal of Sandplay Therapy, 3*(2), 9–12.

Caprio, B. (1989). *The sand tray: An art therapy perspective*. Unpublished master's thesis. Loyola-Marymount University, Los Angeles.

Friedman, H.S. (1986, March). *Sandplay: An approach to the child's unconscious*. Paper presented at the spring lecture series, sponsored by the Hilde Kirsch Children's Center, Los Angeles.

Friedman, H.S., & Mitchell, R.R. (2001). *Survey of therapists who use sandplay therapy attending the International Society of Sandplay Therapy in Zurich, Switzerland*. Unpublished manuscript.

Jung, C.G. (1968). *The collected works of C. G. Jung: Alchemical studies* (Vol. 13, par. 36). Princeton University Press.

Kalff, D. (1980). *Sandplay: A psychotherapeutic approach to the psyche* (W. Ackerman, Trans.). Sigo Press. [Originally published (1966) in German as Sandspiel by Rascher. First published (1971) in English as Sandplay: Mirror of a child's psyche (H. Kirsch, Trans.) by Browser Press].

Kalff, D. (1988). *Sandplay in Switzerland*. Notes of seminar presented at Kalff's home in Zurich, Switzerland, sponsored by the University of California at Santa Cruz.

Miller, R.R. (1979). *Investigation of a psychaotherapeutic tool for adults: The sand tray*. (Doctoral dissertation, California School of Professional Psychology, Fresno). Dissertation Abstracts International 43(1-B): 257. (University Microfilms No. 82-07557).

Perry, J.W. (1973). The creative element in madness. *Art Psychotherapy*, *1*, 61–65.

Weinrib, E.L. (1983). *Images of the self: The sandplay therapy process*. Sigo Press.

Weinrib, E.L. (1989). *Sandplay workshop*. Workshop sponsored by Friends of C.G. Jung, Phoenix, AZ.

Winnicott, D.W. (1965). *The maturational processes and the facilitating environment: Studies in the theory of emotional development*. International Universities Press, Inc. (Originally published in the International Journal of Psycho-Analysis, 39, 416–420).

Chapter 13

Final thoughts

What a wonderful experience it has been for us to revisit the many sandplay scenes our clients created, as well as the teaching we have done throughout the world in the past 40 years. We are grateful to have had these exceptional and profound experiences, especially for the many individuals we have met, shared with, worked with, and taught. As we look back and remember, we know that often we learned more from them than they did from us.

Sandplay has become for both of us a symbolic path that has led us to a deeper expression and understanding of both the conscious and unconscious aspects of the psyche. Discovering nonverbal sandplay work within the context of verbal therapy has opened us to a whole new level of the psyche and an understanding that those images (often intense and sometimes long-forgotten) have emotional effects. Throughout the sandplay process, parts of ourselves are revealed that are not available to verbal methods alone. Sandplay provides a *temenos*, a sacred space for the experience of transformation, essential in this work.

Because of the nonverbal, symbolic experience of expressing spontaneous internal images in the sand and in artwork, we have been profoundly affected by the depths of the psyche that have generated a greater understanding and influence in both our personal as well as our professional lives. One of the functions of sandplay is to give people the space to see aspects of themselves that cannot be known through words. Estelle Weinrib said,

> I believe that the making of a sand picture is in itself a symbolic and creative act, provided it happens within the conditions Kalff called the free and protected space … the symbolic active fantasy by the patient stimulates the imagination. This frees neurotically fixated energy and moves it into creative channels, which in itself can be healing.
>
> (2005, p.23)

We believe sandplay deepens and accelerates the therapeutic endeavor. As the mind and body interact in the sand, the imagination is stimulated and creativity is evoked. While this process is occurring, verbal complexes, dreams, personality, and life problems are thrust toward consciousness. Sandplay encourages a creative regression that enables healing precisely because of delayed interpretation, the silence of the *temenos*, and deliberate discouragement of directed thinking.

We both have been moved to share these sandplay cases and clinical experiences with you. This book is particularly special to us. It is possibly our last opportunity to share our love of sandplay therapy with a broad audience and to share with you some of the most important elements of what we have learned during our sandplay journeys. We hope this book will contribute to your sandplay journey.

We both have come to have a deep respect for the silent essence of the most human relationship that gets established between us as therapist and the individual creating a sandplay. This relationship supports the exploration of unconscious energies and a descent into the depths that sustains the work through the most challenging times. As Jung clearly states, "The inner voice is the voice of a fuller life, of a wider, more comprehensive consciousness" (1954, par.318).

References

1. Jung, C.G. (1954). *The Collected Works of C.G. Jung: Development of personality.* (Vol. 17). Princeton University.
2. Weinrib, E.L. (2005). *Images of the self* (2nd ed.). Temonos Press. (Originally published 1983).

Index

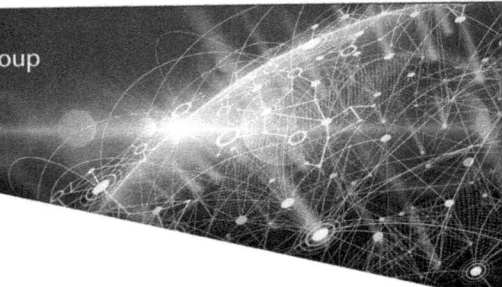

Taylor & Francis Group
an **informa** business

Taylor & Francis eBooks

www.taylorfrancis.com

A single destination for eBooks from Taylor & Francis
with increased functionality and an improved user
experience to meet the needs of our customers.

90,000+ eBooks of award-winning academic content in
Humanities, Social Science, Science, Technology, Engineering,
and Medical written by a global network of editors and authors.

TAYLOR & FRANCIS EBOOKS OFFERS:

A streamlined
experience for
our library
customers

A single point
of discovery
for all of our
eBook content

Improved
search and
discovery of
content at both
book and
chapter level

REQUEST A FREE TRIAL
support@taylorfrancis.com

Routledge
Taylor & Francis Group

CRC Press
Taylor & Francis Group

For Product Safety Concerns and Information please contact our EU
representative GPSR@taylorandfrancis.com
Taylor & Francis Verlag GmbH, Kaufingerstraße 24, 80331 München, Germany

www.ingramcontent.com/pod-product-compliance
Lightning Source LLC
Chambersburg PA
CBHW081738270326
41932CB00020B/3323